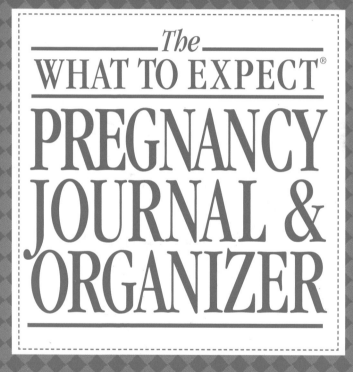

The

WHAT TO EXPECT®

PREGNANCY JOURNAL & ORGANIZER

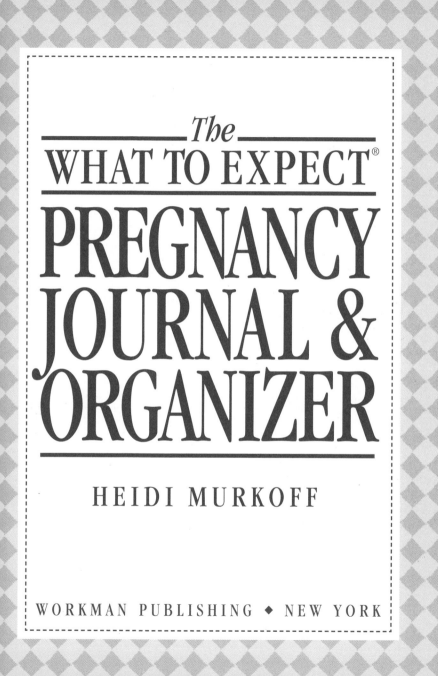

The

WHAT TO EXPECT®

PREGNANCY JOURNAL & ORGANIZER

HEIDI MURKOFF

WORKMAN PUBLISHING ◆ NEW YORK

Copyright © 2006 by What to Expect LLC
WHAT TO EXPECT is a registered trademark of What to Expect LLC.

∼○∼

All rights reserved. No portion of this book may be reproduced—
mechanically, electronically, or by any other means, including
photocopying—without written permission of the publisher.
Published simultaneously in Canada by
Thomas Allen & Son Limited.

ISBN 978-0-7611-4212-6

∼○∼

Book design: Lisa Hollander
Cover design: John Seeger Gilman
Cover mom photograph: © mattbeard.com
Cover quilt: Lynette Parmentier, Quilt Creations
Cover photography: Davies + Starr

Workman books are available at special discounts when purchased
in bulk for premiums and sales promotions as well as for fund-raising
or educational use. Special editions or book excerpts can also be created
to specification. For details, contact the Special Sales Director at the
address below or send an email to specialmarkets@workman.com.

∼○∼

Workman Publishing Co., Inc.
225 Varick Street
New York, NY 10014-4381
workman.com

WORKMAN is a registered trademark of Workman Publishing Co., Inc.

Printed in China
First printing November 2006
21 20 19 18

contents

∽

part two:
my childbirth journal 109

part three:
my pregnancy organizer 135

a place for everything

are you the sentimental sort (and even if you aren't usually, you might be once those hormones start raging)? Or the practical type (and now that you're expecting, you'll have to be—what with all those to-do lists that need doing)? Are you eager to record those special moments you'll never want to forget, from where you were when you found out you were pregnant, to what you were doing when those first contractions hit, to how you felt the first time you cuddled your newborn? Determined to document every detail of your pregnancy and delivery—the symptoms, the test results, the advice your practitioner gave you? Looking for a place to keep track of all your baby business, from childbirth education class notes to practitioner call hours, from medical finances to the layette you'd like to get?

Here's the book that will help you do it all. *The What to Expect Pregnancy Journal & Organizer* is the all-in-one place to write down everything you'll need (and want) to remember about your 40 weeks of baby making.

The first two parts are daily journals—a place for jotting down your feelings, noting your symptoms, chronicling your daily expectant life (and venting about it, too!). And for milestones (Baby's first hiccups! The day your belly button popped!) and memories ("I ate pickle-and-jelly sandwiches every day for three weeks." "Our pet name for baby was 'Pee-Wee.'") Filled out, it'll be a fun keepsake to look back on—a snapshot of 40 amazing weeks that'll be over in a flash, but that you'll always be able to treasure.

The last part is an organizer—a place, well, to keep things organized. Creating (and having) a baby is a miracle, for sure, but it can also be a logistical challenge. Make that *many* logistical challenges. With so many little details that'll demand your attention (Appointments! Test results!), so many decisions that need making (Baby names! Baby cribs!), so many lists that need checking and questions that need asking and celebrations that need planning and thank-you notes that need writing and . . . you get the idea. Log it all in the practical pages of the organizer.

Maybe you'll find the journals are where you spend most of your filling-in hours, maybe you'll live in (and by) the organizer, maybe you'll divide your time—flipping back and forth to cover all your expectant bases. Either way, enjoy keeping track, keeping up, and keeping it all together while you're expecting!

May all your greatest expectations come true! —*Heidi*

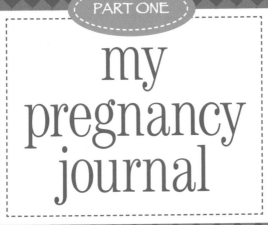

PART ONE

my pregnancy journal

my pregnancy journal

a lot can happen in nine months—and you're about to find that out. Not only will you be making a baby (from scratch) in the 40 weeks that follow, but you'll also be experiencing remarkable changes in your body (good-bye waist, hello breasts!). You'll also be experiencing a range of feelings (from sheer exhilaration to pure terror and back again . . . in 60 seconds) that will bewilder you—and keep your partner on his toes. It'll be a wild ride, but a memorable one—that is, if you write it all down. Use this journal to record everything you'd like to remember about your pregnancy—the crazy symptoms, the wackier emotions, the thrilling moments (and the funny ones and the embarrassing ones), to capture your hopes, your dreams (literally, since they get pretty interesting when you're expecting), your milestones, your memories.

the first month

What I look like this month

[PASTE PICTURE OF YOURSELF HERE]

WAIST SIZE   BRA SIZE

✓ MY TO-DO LIST

Choose a practitioner

Preconception visit. Date _____

Chart ovulation

Begin taking prenatal vitamins

Quit smoking (if applicable)

Quit drinking (if applicable)

Cut down on caffeine

Start eating well (see *What to Expect: Eating Well When You're Expecting*)

Check out health insurance pregnancy coverage

Buy home pregnancy tests (record results on page 14)

memories & milestones

Our thoughts about becoming parents

_____

_____

_____

_____

_____

How I knew I was ovulating

_____

_____

Who we told that we're trying for a baby

_____

_____

_____

We've been trying to conceive for this long

_____

I suspected I might be pregnant because

_____

_____

My partner suspected I might be pregnant because

_____

_____

I'm excited about

_____

_____

_____

_____

I'm nervous about

_____

_____

_____

_____

before you forget

Once the big news is official, record your LMP (last menstrual period) and due date on page 136.

5

HOW I'M FEELING . . .

physically

emotionally

DAY ONE

DAY TWO

DAY THREE

DAY FOUR

the two-week head start

~∞~

You're not even officially pregnant yet, but your pregnancy is officially being counted starting now—two weeks before your baby is even conceived! That's because it's hard to pinpoint the precise moment when sperm meets egg. So in order to give all pregnancies some standard timing, your pregnancy is dated not from conception, but from the first day of your last menstrual period (and that's also where you should begin dating this journal). Which means that by the time your baby is actually conceived, you've already clocked in two weeks of pregnancy (talk about getting a head start)!

DAY FIVE

DAY SIX

DAY SEVEN

NOTES

HOW I'M FEELING . . .

physically

emotionally

DAY ONE

DAY TWO

DAY THREE

DAY FOUR

_____

_____

_____

_____

DAY FIVE

_____

_____

_____

_____

DAY SIX

_____

_____

_____

_____

DAY SEVEN

_____

_____

_____

NOTES _____

_____

_____

_____

tip of the week

start your vitamins

~∞~

It's never too early to start taking care of your baby (even before you conceive!), and the easiest way to start is by popping a prenatal vitamin. Taking a daily prenatal gives you the security of knowing that you're pumped up with all the right baby-making ingredients (including that most essential one, folic acid). And here's another prenatal perk: Taking a daily multivitamin that contains at least 10 mg of vitamin B_6 before conception and during the first few weeks of pregnancy means you're likely to experience fewer episodes of nausea. Who wouldn't want that?

FAST FACT

Congratulations! Though you won't know it yet, this is when you'll conceive your baby!

HOW I'M FEELING . . .

date

physically

emotionally

DAY ONE

DAY TWO

DAY THREE

DAY FOUR

DAY FIVE

DAY SIX

DAY SEVEN

NOTES

HOW I'M FEELING . . .   date

physically

emotionally

DAY ONE

DAY TWO

DAY THREE

DAY FOUR

DAY FIVE

DAY SIX

DAY SEVEN

NOTES

the second month

What I look like
this month

[PASTE PICTURE OF YOURSELF HERE]

WAIST SIZE ___ BRA SIZE ___

MY SYMPTOMS ___

✓ MY TO-DO LIST

Practitioner visit. Date _____

Start keeping a practitioner visit log
(see page 156)

Figure out my due date (record on
page 136)

Schedule early ultrasound,
if recommended. Date _____
(record results on page 152)

the pregnancy test

	DATE	WHERE	BRAND	RESULTS
1st test				
2nd test				
3rd test				

memories & milestones

I found out I was pregnant on

Where I was when I found out

My reaction

Dad's reaction

How I told him

We celebrated by

Who we told (and their reactions)

Foods that make me queasy

Foods I find comforting

Foods I've been craving

I had an early ultrasound on

Our reaction

A message to our baby

Our baby

(PASTE ULTRASOUND PICTURE HERE)

HOW I'M FEELING . . .

date

physically _____

emotionally _____

DAY ONE _____

_____

_____

_____

_____

DAY TWO _____

_____

_____

_____

DAY THREE _____

_____

_____

_____

_____

_____

FAST FACT

By the end of this month, your uterus will be about the size of an orange and your baby will grow from the size of an orange seed to the size of a raspberry. And while you're mulling that tidbit over, peel an orange and enjoy. Citrus fruits (and raspberries, too) are full of baby-friendly vitamin C—plus they're often soothing for the queasy set.

DAY FOUR

DAY FIVE

DAY SIX

DAY SEVEN

NOTES

weighing in

Did you know your prepregnancy weight? If it's been a while since you weighed yourself, you might want to consider stepping on a scale now. That way you'll have a baseline weight from which to calculate your gain during pregnancy (chances are, even with all that bloating you're feeling, you haven't gained much yet). Current guidelines recommend that the average woman gain 25 to 35 pounds over the course of her pregnancy. In this first trimester, you probably won't gain much (a good goal is about 3 or 4 pounds), and if you're really suffering from the queasies, you might even drop a few (that's nothing to worry about this early on—remember, baby's still seed size).

HOW I'M FEELING . . .

date

physically

emotionally

DAY ONE

DAY TWO

DAY THREE

DAY FOUR

it's not easy being green

~∞~

Feeling a little green? Combat that common queasy feeling with ginger. Research shows that this spicy root, long touted as a stomach soother, effectively fights the around-the-clock nausea, or "morning sickness," that can affect you in the first trimester. So brew some ginger tea, toss some chopped fresh ginger into your morning smoothie, shred some into your stir-fry, bake some into carrot-ginger muffins. Or fast-track your ginger: Nibble on crystallized ginger, suck on ginger lollipops or candies, or drink a glass of real ginger ale.

DAY FIVE

DAY SIX

DAY SEVEN

NOTES

HOW I'M FEELING . . .

date

physically

emotionally

DAY ONE

DAY TWO

DAY THREE

DAY FOUR

DAY FIVE

DAY SIX

DAY SEVEN

NOTES

color me safe

Gray doesn't make your day? Not happy about going back to your roots? Check with your practitioner before calling your colorist. Though there's no hard evidence that the chemicals in hair coloring are harmful to your baby, some experts advise waiting out the first trimester before retouching. After that, consider going for highlights instead of single-process color (this way the chemicals won't touch your scalp). You can also ask your colorist about less harsh processing (an ammonia-free base, for instance). And here's something else to consider: Hormonal changes can make your hair react differently, even to your regular formula. Try a test strand before doing your whole head—just to be sure you'll get what you want.

HOW I'M FEELING . . .

physically

emotionally

DAY ONE

the next breast thing

~∽~

You can toss that push-up bra into the back of your closet now—your breasts probably won't need any extra help in the size department during the coming months. In fact, they may already be swelling to proportions you never imagined possible (you might even have grown a full cup size by now). That's all good. But they might also be uncomfortably tender, tingly, and achy (not so good). Try to remember that these changes are for the noble purpose of preparing your breasts for milk production—in other words, your pain is baby's gain. Keep in mind, too, that while your breasts will keep growing, they won't be tender to the touch much longer—sensitivity usually subsides by the end of the first trimester.

DAY TWO

WEEK 8

DAY THREE

DAY FOUR

22

DAY FIVE

DAY SIX

DAY SEVEN

NOTES

the third month

What I look like this month

[PASTE PICTURE OF YOURSELF HERE]

WAIST SIZE _____ BRA SIZE _____

MY SYMPTOMS _____

✓ MY TO-DO LIST

Practitioner visit. Date _____
(fill in practitioner visit log,
 page 156)

Schedule CVS test (if having).
Date _____

Schedule other first-trimester screening.
Date _____

Schedule a dentist appointment.
Date _____

Decide when to spread the news

Go bra shopping

Look into maternity-leave policies at
work

memories & milestones

I first heard my baby's heartbeat on _____

When I heard it, I felt _____

Dad felt _____

24

Our "pet" name for baby

I broke the news at work on

My boss's reaction

My coworkers' reaction

My most exciting pregnancy moment so far

My most embarrassing pregnancy moment so far

My funniest pregnancy moment so far

Foods I can't get enough of

Strangest food I've been craving

Farthest I (or my partner) have gone to satisfy a craving

Foods I can't stand

Smells that make me sick

Highlights of my first trimester

Low points of my first trimester

My message to baby

Dad's message

HOW I'M FEELING . . .

physically

emotionally

DAY ONE

DAY TWO

DAY THREE

FAST FACT

By the end of this month, your uterus will be about the size of a grapefruit and your baby will be the size of a peach. Sounds sweet!

DAY FOUR

DAY FIVE

DAY SIX

DAY SEVEN

NOTES

pickles and ice cream

∾

It's the oldest cliché in the book (and on television sitcoms), but when you're faced with a hankering for honeydew dipped in cream cheese, a longing for lima beans layered with honey and salsa, or a passion for, well, passion fruit, it's no laughing matter. When cravings attack—and when your yen is for something healthy—indulge them. If you're hungering for something that's somewhat lacking in nutritional value (like kettle-cooked potato chips by the vatful, for instance), consider satisfying yourself with a suitable substitute (sliced potatoes, drizzled with olive oil, sprinkled with a little salt and some Parmesan cheese, and baked until crisp).

HOW I'M FEELING . . .

date

physically

emotionally

DAY ONE

_____

_____

_____

_____

_____

DAY TWO

_____

_____

_____

_____

DAY THREE

_____

_____

_____

_____

DAY FOUR

_____

_____

DAY FIVE

DAY SIX

DAY SEVEN

NOTES

do you smell something— or everything?

∽

Can you smell what's on the menu before you even sit down at the table (maybe before you even walk into the restaurant)? Don't worry, you're not turning into a beagle . . . you're just turning into a pregnant woman. Believe it or not, pregnancy hormones cause a super-keen sense of smell—a heightened sensitivity that makes mild odors smell strong, strong odors smell overpowering, and many odors, well, just plain sickening (literally). Since your nose knows all, stay out of stinky restaurants, move your desk chair away from the coworker who's heavy-handed with his cologne, and ask your partner to stay out of sniffing range when he's polishing off a mound of onion rings.

HOW I'M FEELING . . .

physically

emotionally

DAY ONE

DAY TWO

DAY THREE

DAY FOUR

tip of the week
the six-meal solution

∽

When you're pregnant (and hungry), your best offensive is to launch a snack attack. Six mini-meals or snacks a day go a lot further than three squares, keeping blood sugar levels constant and keeping you on the go. Grazing's also the best way to ease the queasies (and that gas). Stock your fridge, pantry, glove compartment, tote bag, purse, desk drawer, and bedside table with plenty of nutritious nibbles: individually wrapped cheese wedges and string cheese; whole-grain granola bars; mini boxes of raisins, cereal, nuts, or trail mix; fresh fruit; dried apricots; soy chips; whole-grain pretzels and crackers; yogurt. Want to keep track of what you're eating? You can start on page 196.

DAY FIVE

DAY SIX

DAY SEVEN

NOTES

HOW I'M FEELING . . .

date

physically

emotionally

DAY ONE

DAY TWO

DAY THREE

DAY FOUR

DAY FIVE

DAY SIX

DAY SEVEN

NOTES

fitness facts

∽

Should you exercise your right to exercise while you're expecting? Absolutely (as long as you have your practitioner's okay). But if it's been a while since you hit the trail (or the pool or the gym), start out slowly. Overdoing it can lead to injury, overheating, nausea (no need for more of that!), and exhaustion (ditto). Plus, if you begin with a bang, you're more likely to go bust—quitting when you're just getting started. A good plan for the pregnant newbie athlete: Begin with ten minutes of gentle warm-up, followed by five minutes of moderately strenuous exercise and a five-minute cool-down. Increase the strenuous segment by five minutes every week until you hit 30 minutes. Keep track of your exercise efforts on page 186.

HOW I'M FEELING . . .

physically

emotionally

DAY ONE

DAY TWO

DAY THREE

DAY FOUR

tip of the week

going oversized

∽

Feeling a little snug around the waist already? No need to rush to the store for maternity clothes just yet. Turn to sweats, yoga pants, tee's, and anything else that stretches; make a fashion statement with billowy blouses, dresses, and skirts; sneak into your partner's closet for oversize shirts; or give your jeans and slacks a new lease on pregnancy life by threading a rubber band through the buttonhole and around the button to allow for your expanding midsection. Low is another way to go (as in wearing pants, skirts, and belts fashionably low—below the belly). When you do head for the store, try not to overdo it. A couple of good-quality maternity skirts, pants, and tops should see you through the next six months. And don't buy ahead—you've got a way to grow!

DAY FIVE

DAY SIX

DAY SEVEN

NOTES

the fourth month

What I look like this month

[PASTE PICTURE OF YOURSELF HERE]

✓ MY TO-DO LIST

Practitioner visit. Date _____
(fill in practitioner visit log, page 156)

Schedule amniocentesis (if having).
Date _____
Record prenatal test results on page 151

Schedule triple/quad screening test.
Date _____

Shop for maternity clothes

WAIST SIZE   BRA SIZE

MY SYMPTOMS

memories & milestones

I started to show on

When I started to show, I felt

When I started wearing maternity clothes, I felt

The nicest thing my partner has said to me

The most annoying thing my partner has said to me

My strangest pregnancy symptoms

Foods I can't get enough of

My prediction of baby's gender

Dad's prediction

My latest exciting pregnancy moment

My latest embarrassing pregnancy moment

My latest funny pregnancy moment

My latest weird pregnancy dream

HOW I'M FEELING . . .

physically

emotionally

DAY ONE

DAY TWO

DAY THREE

FAST FACT

During this month, your baby will grow to about the size of a navel orange, causing your uterus to rise out of the pelvic cavity. Toward the end of the month, you might be able to feel the top of it around two inches below your belly button, if you know what you're feeling for. (Ask your practitioner for some pointers at your next visit.)

DAY FOUR

DAY FIVE

DAY SIX

DAY SEVEN

NOTES

the pound-a-week plan

∽

Weight-wise, your first three months may have been slow going, but now that you're entering your second trimester, let the gain begin. During months four through eight, you'll probably be on the pound-a-week plan— which means you should aim to gain an average of one pound a week (or about four pounds a month). Plot your progress on your weight-gain tracker (see page 217).

HOW I'M FEELING . . .

date

physically

emotionally

DAY ONE

DAY TWO

DAY THREE

DAY FOUR

tip of the week

face facts

More greasy (or blotchy, or pimply) than glowing? Pregnancy hormones can cause your complexion to do some pretty peculiar things. How can you keep your skin looking its best? First, never leave home without applying that sunscreen. Second, continue to moisturize if you're getting dry, but before you reach for any acne cream, make sure it's pregnancy-safe (ask your practitioner)—many aren't. Third, steer clear of perfumed lotions or creams whose added fragrances and chemicals can offend (because of your heightened sense of smell), and irritate (because of your extra-sensitive skin). Finally, treat yourself to a facial (just remember to let your aesthetician know you're expecting).

DAY FIVE

DAY SIX

DAY SEVEN

NOTES

HOW I'M FEELING . . .

physically

emotionally

DAY ONE

WEEK 16

DAY TWO

DAY THREE

DAY FOUR

DAY FIVE

_____

_____

_____

_____

DAY SIX

_____

_____

_____

_____

DAY SEVEN

_____

_____

_____

_____

NOTES

_____

_____

_____

_____

second to none

~∞~

Most expectant women consider their second trimester to be the best of the bunch. That's because early-pregnancy nausea and fatigue have probably passed, and that third-trimester "beached whale" stage hasn't washed over you yet. So while you're enjoying the second trimester's relative smooth sailing, don't just sit there—do the things that you were too queasy and tired to do in your first trimester and may find yourself too bulky and tired to do in your third. Schedule a vacation, plan romantic nights on the town, up your exercise routine, and hit the sheets for some hanky-panky (not necessarily in that order).

HOW I'M FEELING . . .

physically

emotionally

DAY ONE

DAY TWO

DAY THREE

DAY FOUR

WEEK 17

tip of the week

growing is a pain

First the good news: Your uterus has grown large enough that you're actually looking pregnant (instead of like you've been overdoing the ice cream). Now the bad news: Your uterus has grown large enough that it's causing pregnancy growing pains—those achy or sharp pains you sometimes feel on one or both sides of your abdomen. Haven't got time for the pain? Resting in a comfortable position or lying down usually brings at least a little relief from the ache.

DAY FIVE

DAY SIX

DAY SEVEN

NOTES

the fifth month

What I look like this month

[PASTE PICTURE OF YOURSELF HERE]

WAIST SIZE _____ BRA SIZE _____

MY SYMPTOMS _____

_____

_____

_____

_____

✓ **MY TO-DO LIST**

Practitioner visit. Date _____
(fill in practitioner visit log, page 156)

Schedule my level II ultrasound.
Date _____

Decide whether or not to find out
baby's gender at the ultrasound
(record ultrasound and other prenatal
test results on pages 151–155)

Shop for maternity clothes

memories & milestones

I felt my baby move on _____

It felt like _____

How I felt _____

When I saw baby on the ultrasound, I felt _____

Dad felt

During the ultrasound, we found out that we're having a

When I found out, I felt

Dad felt

We decided not to find out baby's gender because

I hope our baby has my

I hope our baby has Dad's

My message to our baby

Dad's message

My latest weird dream

What I like best about being pregnant

What I like least about being pregnant

Friends and family who are pregnant and when they're due

Our baby

(PASTE ULTRASOUND PICTURE HERE)

HOW I'M FEELING . . .

date

physically

emotionally

DAY ONE

DAY TWO

DAY THREE

(FAST FACT)

At 20 weeks, your baby will be the size of a small cantaloupe and the top of your uterus will reach your belly button. By the end of the month, your uterus will be about an inch above your belly button.

DAY FOUR

DAY FIVE

DAY SIX

DAY SEVEN

NOTES

can't get enough of it

~∽~

Sex, sex, and more sex. With first-trimester queasiness and fatigue a thing of the past (hopefully), you might find yourself with a libido that just won't quit. You can thank hormonal changes—and the increased blood flow to your pelvic region—for this sexual revolution. On top (so to speak) of that are the new curves and larger-than-life breasts that you're sporting now—perhaps making you feel more sensuous, sultry, and sexy than ever. If that sounds like you, and red light activities have been green-lighted by your practitioner, embrace your desire (and your partner). And even if he's exhausted by your sexual shenanigans, encourage him to play along—because the clock is ticking. Many couples find their libido leaves the bedroom as soon as a new-born moves in. Not in the mood for love? That's normal, too—pregnancy affects dif-ferent women different ways.

HOW I'M FEELING . . .

date

physically

emotionally

DAY ONE

DAY TWO

DAY THREE

DAY FOUR

tip of the week

yoga baby

Yoga is a perfect exercise for the pregnant body and soul. It emphasizes breathing, relaxation, posture, and body awareness, and it can help build strength, increase endurance, improve alignment, and reduce aches and pains. Can't connect with your inner lotus position? Join a pregnancy Pilates class. Pilates can help stretch and loosen your spine, plus it can release tension. Just be sure *any* exercise you do (including yoga and Pilates) is specifically designed for the pregnant set.

DAY FIVE

DAY SIX

DAY SEVEN

NOTES

HOW I'M FEELING . . .

date

physically

emotionally

DAY ONE

DAY TWO

DAY THREE

DAY FOUR

DAY FIVE

DAY SIX

DAY SEVEN

NOTES

tip of the week

buckle up

∞

Wondering how you're supposed to buckle in your ever-growing belly? To travel safely when you're expecting, make sure the lap belt is under your expanding abdomen and across your hips (it should be lying over your pelvis) and place the shoulder belt between your breasts. Remember, the best way to keep your baby safe is to protect yourself.

HOW I'M FEELING . . .

physically

emotionally

DAY ONE

DAY TWO

DAY THREE

DAY FOUR

tip of the week

shape up before baby ships out

Maybe you've never thought much about your pelvic muscles—or maybe you never even realized you had any. But it's time to pay attention now. They'll need to stretch during delivery (baby's got a big head, after all), and they'll need to tighten up after you give birth. The good news about pelvic strengthening exercises—called Kegels—is that you can do them anywhere (at your desk, while driving, while in line at the store, while making love). All you have to do is tighten, hold (for at least five seconds), and then release the muscles that you use to stop the stream of urine when you pee. If you feel your stomach tensing or your thighs or buttocks contracting, you're working the wrong muscles.

DAY FIVE

DAY SIX

DAY SEVEN

NOTES

HOW I'M FEELING . . .

physically

emotionally

DAY ONE

DAY TWO

DAY THREE

DAY FOUR

DAY FIVE

_____

_____

_____

_____

DAY SIX

_____

_____

_____

_____

DAY SEVEN

_____

_____

_____

_____

NOTES

_____

_____

_____

_____

big foot?

Check out your feet. Notice anything different about them? If you're like many moms-to-be, you'll find that they're growing along with your uterus (though not as fast, fortunately). That's because the pregnancy hormone that loosens the ligaments and joints in your pelvis (so that your baby can fit through) also loosens the ligaments and joints in the rest of your body, including your feet, causing foot bones to spread. The result? Your shoe size may increase a half or whole size, making you feel less the Little Mama and more the Big Foot. Unlike your belly, which will (hopefully) return to its original size soon after delivery, your feet may not— good news if you'd like an excuse to go shoe shopping. In the meantime, accommodate your growing tootsies by buying shoes that are sensible, comfortable, and roomy enough—and save the stilettos for later.

the sixth month

What I look like this month

[PASTE PICTURE OF YOURSELF HERE]

WAIST SIZE   BRA SIZE

MY SYMPTOMS

✓ MY TO-DO LIST

Practitioner visit. Date _____
(fill in practitioner visit log, page 156)

Schedule my glucose screening test.
Date _____

Sign up for childbirth preparation
classes (record class notes on page 220)

Start browsing for baby gear
(keep track on page 245)

Think about baby names (jot down
possibilities on page 243)

memories 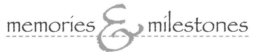 milestones

Baby's movements feel like

Baby is most active during

I first felt baby hiccup on

My belly button popped on

How I feel about my body now

What I miss most about my non-pregnant body

Forgetful moments I've had recently

Best pregnancy advice I've gotten

Strangest pregnancy advice I've gotten

Some things about pregnancy that have surprised me

Some things I wish someone had told me about pregnancy

Nicest thing a stranger has said/done

Rudest thing a stranger has said/done

What I'm most looking forward to about motherhood

What makes me nervous about being a mother

My message to baby

Dad's message

HOW I'M FEELING . . .

date

physically

emotionally

DAY ONE

DAY TWO

DAY THREE

FAST FACT

As you reach the two-thirds mark of your pregnancy, your baby weighs around two pounds and your uterus reaches about two and a half inches above your belly button (a belly button that, as you've probably noticed, has taken on a life of its own . . . popping up like the timer on a Thanksgiving turkey).

DAY FOUR

DAY FIVE

DAY SIX

DAY SEVEN

NOTES

a hairy situation

‿∽

Feeling a little ape-like these days, what with all the hair you're suddenly sprouting in places you'd rather not, including your face, back, and stomach? Chin up (if you dare). This hormonally triggered hairy situation is—thankfully—only temporary, and delivery will bring an end to it. Even so, it's probably best to skip popular hair-removal treatments (such as lasers, electrolysis, and depilatories) until after you give birth. Ditto for lightening treatments and bleaching. While no studies have been done to determine for sure whether they're harmful or not, it's certainly better to be safe (and hairy) than sorry. But do keep those tweezers, shavers, and waxing kits handy. There's nothing wrong with plucking, pulling off, or shaving during your nine months (just be extra careful, since your skin is extra sensitive).

HOW I'M FEELING . . .

physically

emotionally

DAY ONE

DAY TWO

DAY THREE

DAY FOUR

DAY FIVE

DAY SIX

DAY SEVEN

NOTES

boning up on calcium

~

While drinking milk might be the most obvious way to bone up on calcium (vital for building those cute little baby bones and baby teeth—and for protecting your own bone density), it's far from the only way. If it doesn't appeal straight up, hide the white stuff in your smoothies or creamy soups and cereal (select lactose-free milk if your tummy's finicky). Or bypass the milk case entirely and choose dairy products that won't leave a sour taste in your mouth—yogurt and cheese, for instance. Actually, there's really no need to visit the dairy department at all to score your calcium fix. You'll find calcium in fortified fruit juice, calcium-enriched soy milk, tofu, dark leafy greens, broccoli, and canned salmon. Keep track of your calcium intake (and all your Daily Dozen) starting on page 196.

HOW I'M FEELING . . .

physically

emotionally

DAY ONE

DAY TWO

DAY THREE

DAY FOUR

DAY FIVE

_____

DAY SIX

_____

DAY SEVEN

_____

NOTES

beauty and the pregnancy beast

ꝏ

Not loving the skin you're in since pregnancy hormones started calling the shots (and the blotches and the pimples and the irritation)? Try a little makeup magic. A good concealer can hide those blemishes and discolorations, and a natural bronzer or pinkish blush can give you that glow you thought you were supposed to have. Is your nose starting to spread (like everything else on your body)? Slim it down by dotting some concealer along the sides and brushing a light shade of blush or bronzer down the center of it. Can't find your cheekbones anymore? Apply a light shade of blush to the apples of your cheeks (those should be easy to locate these days) and a slightly deeper shade along the line of your cheekbones (where they used to be, at least) and then blend. You glow, girl!

HOW I'M FEELING . . .

physically

emotionally

DAY ONE

DAY TWO

DAY THREE

DAY FOUR

tip of the week

dream, dream, dream

∽

Pregnancy's a dream—make that many dreams, played in rapid succession. Daydreams, nightmares, happy dreams, nervous dreams, sexy dreams, sappy dreams, dreams that border on the bizarre, dreams so vivid they seemed to be recorded in HD, you name it. If you're pregnant, you're dreaming—day and night. Don't lose any sleep over your dreams—they're completely normal (even when they seem completely crazy). But do write them down— they'll be fascinating to look back at one day.

DAY FIVE

DAY SIX

DAY SEVEN

NOTES

HOW I'M FEELING . . .

date

physically

emotionally

DAY ONE

DAY TWO

DAY THREE

DAY FOUR

DAY FIVE

_____

_____

_____

DAY SIX

_____

_____

_____

DAY SEVEN

_____

_____

_____

_____

NOTES

_____

_____

_____

_____

tip of the week

heart (rate) of gold

∽

When you're exercising during pregnancy, keep in mind that your heart is pumping for two. Which means you need to keep twice as close an eye on your heart rate. Happily, you don't have to take your pulse to check the rate (who can find it anyway?). Instead, use the exercise-talk test to see if you're exerting yourself too much. If you can't exercise and talk at the same time (no need to chew gum, too), your heart rate is probably too high. That's your hint to slow it down.

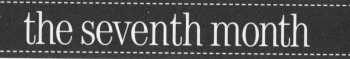

the seventh month

WELCOME TO THE THIRD TRIMESTER

What I look like this month

[PASTE PICTURE OF YOURSELF HERE]

WAIST SIZE   BRA SIZE

MY SYMPTOMS

✓ MY TO-DO LIST

Practitioner visit. Date _____
(fill in practitioner visit log, page 156)

Attend childbirth preparation classes
(record class notes on page 220)

Start shopping for baby gear (keep track
on page 245)

Begin interviewing pediatricians, birth
doulas, baby nurses, or postpartum
doulas (see pages 237, 266, and 268)

Read up on breastfeeding

Do daily kick counts
(keep track on page 218)

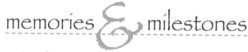

memories & milestones

My baby is most active when

My baby's kicks feel like

70

The first time I saw baby's kicks

The first time I saw baby's hiccups

My appetite has been

The foods I've been craving

Foods that give me heartburn

A recent forgetful moment

My clumsiest pregnancy moment

My funniest pregnancy experience

My most embarrassing pregnancy experience

A recent dream

A recent daydream

When I close my eyes and think of baby, I see

Some things I wish for my baby

My message to baby

Dad's message

HOW I'M FEELING . . .

date

physically

emotionally

DAY ONE

DAY TWO

DAY THREE

(FAST FACT)

By the end of this month, your uterus can be felt four inches above your belly button (or what used to be your belly button . . .) and your baby will weigh in at three pounds.

DAY FOUR

DAY FIVE

DAY SIX

DAY SEVEN

NOTES

forget about it!

~∞~

You're probably having a memorable pregnancy—the only problem is, you can't remember any of it. Forget to pick up the dry cleaning—again? Miss yet another important meeting? Misplace your cell phone for the third time in three hours? Blame hormonally induced pregnancy forgetfulness (fondly nicknamed "placenta brain"). Writing down as much as possible in this book will help keep you focused. So will keeping a pad, pen, and Post-its in strategic places. Or making sure you keep your smartphone up-to-date. And because it takes a village to keep a pregnant woman on task, enlist those around you to serve as your memory backup (have a colleague e-mail you half an hour before the meeting starts). Above all, try to keep your sense of humor—pregnancy forgetfulness will last only as long as your pregnancy.

my bed rest

⁓

Has your practitioner sent you to bed? Whether it's for a few days or a few months, you'll have plenty of time on your hands to fill in this journal (or write a book . . . or two). Put the details about your bed rest down here—and your feelings about it, too.

I was put on bed rest on

Because

For how long?

My reaction

Dad's reaction

I'm keeping myself busy by

Web sites I've been visiting

Movies I've watched

Books I've read _____

_____

_____

The best thing about bed rest _____

_____

The worst thing about bed rest _____

_____

What I miss most _____

_____

_____

What I miss least _____

_____

_____

Some of my visitors _____

_____

The nicest thing my partner has done for me _____

_____

The nicest thing someone else has done for me _____

_____

Notes _____

_____

_____

_____

_____

_____

HOW I'M FEELING . . .

date

physically

emotionally

DAY ONE

DAY TWO

DAY THREE

DAY FOUR

DAY FIVE

_____

DAY SIX

_____

DAY SEVEN

_____

NOTES

every kick counts

$\sim$

Baby's kicking up a storm, but are you keeping count? You should be now that you've passed your 28th week. Twice a day, lie down (as if you need an excuse to rest) or sit quietly at your desk, and count the number of kicks, nudges, pokes, twists, rolls, and other movements your baby makes. You're looking for at least ten movements in an hour's time to be sure your baby's doing just fine. Not getting to ten? Take a drink of something sweet—OJ for instance—and count again. Still not getting ten? Not to worry (baby might be taking a long nap), but do call your practitioner to be sure if you haven't gotten ten kicks in a two-hour test period. Keep track of your daily kick counts on page 218.

HOW I'M FEELING . . .

date

physically

emotionally

DAY ONE

DAY TWO

DAY THREE

DAY FOUR

tip of the week

walk the walk

∽

As long as your practitioner has given you the go-ahead, there's no good reason to quit exercising now. In fact, exercise in the third trimester is one of the best ways to feel your best, and it even combats the fatigue that's been planting you on the sofa in the first place. Plus, it helps get you (or keep you) in shape for the Iron Woman competition that's around the corner: childbirth. Getting that exercise is as easy as taking a walk. Walking is the perfect third-trimester work-out—it's easy on your knees and ankles, it gets your heart revving, and the side-to-side sway of your hips (you call it "waddling") may ease your baby's head into your pelvis, giving you a leg up on labor when the time comes. So walk the walk, Mama!

DAY FIVE

DAY SIX

DAY SEVEN

NOTES

HOW I'M FEELING . . .

physically

emotionally

DAY ONE

DAY TWO

DAY THREE

DAY FOUR

DAY FIVE

DAY SIX

DAY SEVEN

NOTES

sleeping like a baby—not!

∞

The phrase "snooze or lose" is taking on a whole new meaning for you lately—and you're coming out the loser. Ironically (and unfairly), just when you need your sleep the most, you can't seem to get it. To entice the sandman into your bed at night, get your exercise, but get it early in the day—no later than a couple of hours before turning in. Ditto for dinner (though a light snack—a carrot muffin and warm milk, or cheese and crackers—can keep midnight munchies from waking you). Keep your late evenings as stress-free as a pregnant woman possibly can (try to empty your mind), and top off your bedtime routine with a warm bath. Listen to soothing music, grab a book, or grab your partner for some loving until drowsiness sets in. If sleep still eludes you, think of it this way: At least you'll be prepared for the sleepless nights ahead!

the eighth month

What I look like this month

[PASTE PICTURE OF YOURSELF HERE]

WAIST SIZE   BRA SIZE

MY SYMPTOMS

✓ **MY TO-DO LIST**

Practitioner visit. Date _____
(fill in practitioner visit log, page 156)

Attend childbirth preparation classes
(record class notes on page 220)

Schedule an infant CPR class.
Date _____

Put together a birth plan (see page 228)

Do daily kick counts (keep track on
page 218)

Think about cord blood banking

Discuss newborn screening tests with
your practitioner

Tour a hospital/birthing center.
Date _____ (for questions to
ask see page 225)

Shower time! (record it all on page 257)

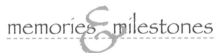

memories & milestones

Baby's latest moves

I felt my first Braxton-Hicks on

Besides the obvious, this part of my body is swollen, too

How I'm feeling about my body

How I'm feeling in general

My most recent clumsy moment

Recently I dreamed

The best pregnancy advice I've gotten lately

The worst pregnancy advice I've gotten lately

I'm most sick of hearing

The nicest thing my partner has said to me

The nicest thing my partner has done for me

What I'll miss the most about being pregnant

What I'll miss the least

What I'm looking forward to the most about becoming a mom

My message to baby

Dad's message

HOW I'M FEELING . . .

date

physically

emotionally

DAY ONE

DAY TWO

DAY THREE

FAST FACT

By this month, your baby's weighing in at five pounds and the measurement in centimeters from the top of your pubic bone to the top of your uterus is roughly equivalent
to the number of weeks of pregnancy. If you ever forget what week you're in (as if!), just
pull out the tape measure and check your progress.

DAY FOUR

DAY FIVE

DAY SIX

DAY SEVEN

NOTES

when you're benched

~∞~

Don't be a working stiff. If you spend much of your day sitting at a desk, make sure you get up for frequent stretching breaks. And don't just sit there when you're just sitting there, either. Next time you're stuck in your chair, try these exercises: Extend your legs, flex your feet, and wiggle your toes while taking a few deep breaths. Next, flex your neck by tilting your head to one side without raising your shoulders (try to "melt" them down instead). Hold for three seconds and exhale. Repeat on the other side. Then, turn from side to side, slowly twisting at the waist, keeping your arms bent at your sides. Finally, clench your butt and hold for a count of two, then release. Repeat a few times. And don't forget that anytime/ anywhere exercise: Kegels.

HOW I'M FEELING . . .

physically

emotionally

DAY ONE

DAY TWO

DAY THREE

DAY FOUR

DAY FIVE

DAY SIX

DAY SEVEN

NOTES

everything's going swell here

~∞~

Sure your belly is swelling, but what's up with the swelling you're noticing in your feet, ankles, and hands, too? Feeling like the Goodyear Blimp may not be so swell, but mild swelling is completely normal —and completely temporary. The best way to minimize pregnancy puff is to drink lots of water (the more you drink, the less you retain). Also avoid sitting or standing for long periods, and rest with your feet elevated. The good news, Puff Mommy: You'll deflate completely soon after you give birth.

HOW I'M FEELING . . .

physically

emotionally

DAY ONE

DAY TWO

DAY THREE

DAY FOUR

tip of the week

it's a date

Sure, you're about to become a couple of parents—but that doesn't mean you should stop thinking of yourselves as a couple. Keeping your relationship front-and-center will keep your baby-to-be from coming between you (though right now, your belly almost certainly will). Nurture your twosome by instituting a weekly date, and consider continuing your romantic ritual after baby makes three (though during those newborn weeks, you may be taking those dates at home).

WEEK 34

DAY FIVE

DAY SIX

DAY SEVEN

NOTES

HOW I'M FEELING . . .   date

physically

emotionally

DAY ONE

DAY TWO

DAY THREE

DAY FOUR

DAY FIVE

DAY SIX

DAY SEVEN

NOTES

relax, baby

With D-day fast approaching, and with so many things to get done before baby moves out of your uterus and into your home, you're probably doing a lot more running around than relaxing. But don't forget to take time for R&R while you still have the time (reality check: as a new mom, you won't). Loosen up those tense muscles and soothe those strained nerves (and prebaby jitters) by taking a relaxation break. A day at the spa and a prenatal massage isn't in the (credit) cards right now? Try this instead: Tense your facial muscles for five seconds, then slowly relax them. Do the same with your neck muscles, then your shoulders, working your way down your body. Don't forget to relax each muscle group before moving on to the next. Keep your breathing deep and slow.

the ninth month

AND BEYOND!

What I look like this month

[PASTE PICTURE OF YOURSELF HERE]

DATE

WAIST SIZE   BRA SIZE

MY SYMPTOMS

✓ MY TO-DO LIST

Practitioner visits. Dates _____
(fill in practitioner visit log, page 156)

Schedule group B strep test.
Date _____

Pack a hospital or birthing-center bag
(see page 239)

Pick out birth announcements

Write up a birth announcement list
(see page 261)

Finish baby shopping

Do daily kick counts
(keep track on page 218)

Do perineal massage

Do a thorough grocery shopping

Stock the freezer with ready-cooked
meals

Find out which restaurants deliver

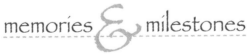

memories & milestones

How I'm feeling these days _____

Baby's kicks feel like _____

I'm having Braxton-Hicks this often

The best advice I've gotten about labor

The worst advice I've gotten about labor

What I wish people would stop telling me about labor

What about childbirth excites me

What about childbirth makes me nervous

My craziest "nesting" moments

I began my maternity leave on

Before I left work, my colleagues did this for me

Predictions about baby's hair color

Predictions about baby's eye color

I predict I'll go into labor on   Dad predicts

Things I've done to try to bring on labor

My message to baby

Dad's message

For labor and delivery memories, see page 123

HOW I'M FEELING . . .

physically

emotionally

DAY ONE

DAY TWO

DAY THREE

DAY FOUR

DAY FIVE

DAY SIX

DAY SEVEN

NOTES

a drop in the bucket... on the floor...

∽

Are you the not-so-proud owner of ten thumbs and two left feet these days? Are you dropping (and breaking) everything you pick up? Bumping into everything (and everyone) in your path? There are plenty of reasons why you're an expectant klutz, from lack of balance thanks to your ever-swelling belly to the loosening of your joints and ligaments, which makes it harder to keep a firm grasp on objects . . . and a lot easier to lose your grip. Your best bets in the fight against the clumsies? Slow down, walk more carefully, avoid pushing yourself to the point of fatigue, and use your brain (if that's still working) when it comes to safety: Steer clear of ice patches, don't climb ladders, let other people do the heavy lifting, and hold on tight to the handrails. And don't pick up anything you'd rather not break!

HOW I'M FEELING . . .

date

physically

emotionally

DAY ONE

DAY TWO

DAY THREE

FAST FACT

Your pregnancy—and your baby—is considered full term once you hit the 37th week. Of course, that doesn't mean baby got the memo—or that he or she will be arriving any time soon. Lots of babies (especially firstborns) opt to overstay their nine-month welcome. Month ten, anyone?

DAY FOUR

DAY FIVE

DAY SIX

DAY SEVEN

NOTES

feathering your nest?

∽

Wait, wasn't it just last week when you didn't have the strength to make a to-do list, never mind do anything on it? So why, all of a sudden, do you have the energy and ambition and endurance of twelve (nonpregnant) women? Why are you suddenly cleaning out closets you forgot you had? Scrubbing grout lines with a toothbrush? Alphabetizing the contents of your fridge? Chalk it up to nesting, that very common compulsion to clean house (and "feather your nest") before baby arrives.

If it strikes you (some moms find the sofa never loses its appeal in late pregnancy), let it run (and clean) its course. But don't get carried away. Nest with common sense (let daddy-to-be paint the baby's room, don't inhale too much of those household-cleaner fumes, and watch your back when you're bending over to scrub). And remember to save up some energy for the Big Event.

HOW I'M FEELING . . .

date

physically

emotionally

DAY ONE

DAY TWO

DAY THREE

DAY FOUR

labor and delivery food?

∽

Should all food be off the table once labor begins? Though some practitioners still recommend a hunger strike once the contractions strike, many now say fine to food, especially in the early stages of labor. In fact, research shows that labor is shorter—as much as 45 to 90 minutes shorter—in women who are allowed eating privileges. If you're given the gastronomic green light, skip the steak and graze your way lightly through labor on foods that are especially easy to digest: broth, toast with jam, plain pasta, applesauce, Jell-O, sorbet, Popsicles. If you can't face food or it's off-limits, there's always the good old labor standby—sucking on ice chips. Make your coach the Ice Man and make sure the ice cometh often.

DAY FIVE

DAY SIX

DAY SEVEN

NOTES

HOW I'M FEELING . . .

physically

emotionally

DAY ONE

DAY TWO

DAY THREE

DAY FOUR

tip of the week

sprung a leak?

Worried about springing a leak now that labor's right around the corner? Here's the good news: Contrary to popular pregnancy belief, more than 85 percent of women will not (repeat: will not) break their "bag of waters," or amniotic sac, before labor begins. Here's even more good news: If you're among those few who do, you don't have to worry about localized flooding at your feet. Amniotic fluid is more likely to come out as a slow leak, a trickle, or a small gush.

DAY FIVE

DAY SIX

DAY SEVEN

NOTES

HOW I'M FEELING . . .   date

physically

emotionally

DAY ONE

DAY TWO

DAY THREE

DAY FOUR

DAY FIVE

DAY SIX

DAY SEVEN

NOTES

giving mother nature a nudge

∞

Tired of waiting? Want to give Mother Nature a little kick in the pants (or a big one)? Many women swear by such do-it-yourself labor inducers as walking, having sex, or even eating spicy food. There's no harm in trying these at home, though if you're looking for scientific evidence that'll prove their effectiveness, you'll be hard-pressed to find any. Looking for labor in a cup of black cohosh or raspberry leaf tea, or a shot of castor oil? They might be just what your grandmother ordered, but not necessarily your practitioner (check first about safety). A foot massage may kick-start labor, but you'll need to know exactly where to rub (put yourself in the hands of a professional reflexologist or ask your practitioner for tips). Bottom line: You can coax all you want to, but chances are your baby won't arrive until he or she is good and ready to arrive.

weeks 41 to 42

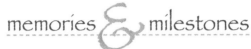

memories & milestones

HOW I'M FEELING . . .

physically

emotionally

I hate/love being overdue because

Advice I've gotten for starting labor

Things I've tried to get labor started

DAY ONE

DAY TWO

WEEK 41

DAY THREE

DAY FOUR

DAY FIVE

DAY SIX

DAY SEVEN

lady in waiting ... and waiting

∽

Got baby on the brain? It's hard to think about anything else when your due date has come and gone. Try to keep your mind off your tardy baby by keeping yourself busy. Use these last few pre-baby days as a time to pamper yourself (it'll be a while before you have that chance again). Treat yourself to a blow-dry (your hair will be less likely to get tangled during labor if it's freshly coiffed), get a mani, a pedi, or a facial (or all three), get waxed (since shaving's probably been out of reach for a while now), go to a movie and dinner with a gal pal, or spend a romantic night out on the town with your partner. You deserve it.

How I'm feeling . . .

date

physically

emotionally

DAY ONE

DAY TWO

DAY THREE

DAY FOUR

DAY FIVE

DAY SIX

DAY SEVEN

NOTES

NOTES

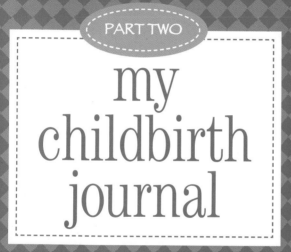

PART TWO

my
childbirth
journal

my childbirth journal

You've been pregnant for nine months (give or take), and the only thing that stands between you and the baby you've been waiting to hold is labor and delivery. It'll be over before you know it (though it may sometimes seem as if it'll never be over, especially somewhere around 6 centimeters' dilation)—but you'll want to remember it forever. To make sure you'll be able to, use this Childbirth Journal to record every moment.

i'm in prelabor

is your body revving up its labor engine, getting ready for the big event? If so, you may notice some of these prelabor symptoms. (Then again, some bodies—especially experienced ones—go about getting ready for labor more quietly, and you may not notice any prelabor signs. That's normal, too).

MY BABY DROPPED ON | date

I BEGAN TO LOSE WEIGHT ON | date

I GOT A BURST OF ENERGY ON | date

I LOST MY MUCOUS PLUG ON | date

I NOTICED BLOODY SHOW ON | date

MY WATER BROKE ON | date

i'm in labor

ready or not, it's show time. You're in labor, which means baby's debut is just around the corner. While you still can write (things might get a little shaky down the line) and still remember (they're sure to be a blur later), record how this momentous event began.

My contractions started on

At this time

They were this far apart

They lasted this long

They felt like
_____

I knew it was really labor because
_____

When the contractions started, I was here
_____

I was doing this
_____

I was with
_____

The weather was
_____

The last thing I ate was
_____

When I realized I was in labor, I felt
_____

Other symptoms
_____

I contacted my partner at
_____

His reaction
_____

I called my practitioner at
_____

I received the following instructions
_____

I passed the time at home by
_____

I left for the hospital or birthing center at
_____

I went by
_____

People who came with me
_____

NOTES
_____

my contraction record

Why record your contractions? First of all, because it'll give you—and your practitioner—a better sense of your progress (and where you're at, labor-wise). Also because when it's all said, done, and delivered, you'll want to look back and relive your baby's arrival into the world (minus the pain, that is).

I'm in labor

[PASTE PICTURE OF YOURSELF HERE]

TIME STARTS	DURATION	TIME STARTS	DURATION

TIME NOW

HOW FAR APART ARE CONTRACTIONS NOW (FROM START TO START)?

HOW LONG DOES EACH LAST (FROM START TO FINISH)?

NOTES

TIME STARTS	DURATION	TIME STARTS	DURATION

TIME NOW

HOW FAR APART ARE CONTRACTIONS NOW (FROM START TO START)?

HOW LONG DOES EACH LAST (FROM START TO FINISH)?

NOTES

TIME STARTS	DURATION	TIME STARTS	DURATION

TIME NOW

HOW FAR APART ARE CONTRACTIONS NOW (FROM START TO START)?

HOW LONG DOES EACH LAST (FROM START TO FINISH)?

NOTES

TIME STARTS	DURATION	TIME STARTS	DURATION

TIME NOW

HOW FAR APART ARE CONTRACTIONS NOW (FROM START TO START)?

HOW LONG DOES EACH LAST (FROM START TO FINISH)?

NOTES

TIME STARTS	DURATION	TIME STARTS	DURATION

TIME NOW

HOW FAR APART ARE CONTRACTIONS NOW (FROM START TO START)?

HOW LONG DOES EACH LAST (FROM START TO FINISH)?

NOTES

TIME STARTS	DURATION	TIME STARTS	DURATION

TIME NOW

HOW FAR APART ARE CONTRACTIONS NOW (FROM START TO START)?

HOW LONG DOES EACH LAST (FROM START TO FINISH)?

NOTES

TIME STARTS	DURATION	TIME STARTS	DURATION

TIME NOW

HOW FAR APART ARE CONTRACTIONS NOW (FROM START TO START)?

HOW LONG DOES EACH LAST (FROM START TO FINISH)?

NOTES

my labor and delivery journal

f rom first contraction to last push, here's the place to record every detail of your labor and delivery (even the parts you might want to forget).

first stage: labor

First (Early or Latent) Phase of Labor
(contractions 5–20 minutes apart; cervix 0–3 cm. dilated)

First phase began

How I felt physically

How I felt emotionally

I arrived at the hospital/birthing center at

When I arrived, here's what happened

My labor nurse(s)

My room number is

Here's what my room looked like

Who was with me

What I ate

What I drank

What I did between contractions

Medical interventions, if any (IV, fetal monitoring, etc.)

NOTES

Second (Active) Phase of Labor
(contractions 3–4 minutes apart; cervix 3–7 cm. dilated)

Second phase began

How many hours from beginning of labor?

How I felt physically

How I felt emotionally

I managed the pain of labor by

Who was with me

My labor nurse(s)

What I did between contractions

Medical interventions, if any (IV, fetal monitoring, etc.)

NOTES

Third (Active or Transitional) Phase of Labor
(contractions 2–3 minutes apart, 60–90 seconds long; cervix 7–10 cm. dilated)

Third phase began

How many hours from beginning of labor?

How I felt physically

How I felt emotionally

I managed the pain of labor by

Who was with me

My labor nurse(s)

What I did between contractions

Medical interventions, if any (IV, fetal monitoring, etc.)

- -

Labor Interventions

The anesthesia or medication I received during labor was

After receiving the medication, I felt

My labor was induced by

How I felt

My labor was helped along by

How I felt

NOTES

second stage: delivery

Vaginal Delivery

I began pushing at

I pushed in these positions

I pushed for this long

How I felt physically

How I felt emotionally

Pain relief, if any

Medical interventions, if any

Complications, if any

Who else was at the delivery?

Their reactions

Who cut the cord?

NOTES

Surgical Delivery

The reason for the C-section

Who was in the room with me

How I felt physically

How I felt emotionally

What the C-section felt like

What I was able to see

It took this long

Anesthesia used

How long I was in recovery

NOTES

- -

The Birth

My baby was born at

My baby was delivered by

How I felt physically

How I felt emotionally

How my partner felt

Did baby cry right away?

I was able to hold my baby

How I felt

I breastfed my baby

How I felt

The placenta was delivered at

Cord blood was banked

Other highlights

Who went with the baby to the nursery

NOTES

labor memories

The hardest part of labor and delivery was

The best part was

The most unexpected part was

The funniest part was

The nicest things my partner did for me

The nicest thing my partner said to me

The dumbest thing my partner did or said to me

How I felt during my labor and delivery

How I felt afterward

My message to baby

Dad's message

NOTES

my baby is born!

after nine months of waiting, and more hours of labor than you might care to recall (or repeat), your baby is finally in your arms instead of in your belly. Jot down all the news about baby's arrival that's fit to print here.

My baby was born on this day

At this time

The weather was

Local and national events in the news

MY BABY'S WEIGHT

LENGTH

HEAD CIRCUMFERENCE

CHEST CIRCUMFERENCE

MY BABY'S APGAR SCORE AT 1 MINUTE

MY BABY'S APGAR AT 5 MINUTES

The results of my baby's first physical exam

Other tests/test results

_____

_____

_____

Other procedures

_____

before you forget

Remember to let your health insurance company know that you've given birth. That way your baby will be covered by your insurance right from the start (it doesn't happen automatically).

meet my baby

a ll that hard work has paid off—and you've just been handed the cuddly payoff! As you hold that precious bundle and gaze into that little face for the first time, you're bound to want to soak it all in. Once you've soaked, detail your first glimpse of baby here.

Baby's name

Baby is named for

We chose this name because

Baby's nickname (if any)

Baby's hair color   How much hair

Baby's eye color

Baby looks like

Baby has Mom's

Baby has Dad's

Baby's birthmarks

Dimples and little folds that merit mention

Baby was born with (check those applicable)

- ☐ lanugo
- ☐ vernix
- ☐ cone-shaped head
- ☐ folded ear
- ☐ other

The first thing I noticed about my baby

The thing that most surprised me about my baby's appearance

Our first meeting

[PLACE FIRST PHOTO HERE]

fabulous firsts

i n the months—and years—to come, there will be hundreds of firsts for your baby (and for you!). But the first firsts are the ones you'll always want to remember. Write them down here.

First meeting with sibling(s)

First meeting with grandparent(s)

First meeting with other family members

First visitors

My baby's first feeding experience

My baby's first poop

my hospital/
birthing center stay

there's no happier place in a hospital than the labor and delivery wing. Though you may not be entirely happy the whole time you're there (women in labor rarely are!), you'll still want to remember everything about your stay, from checking in (pregnant) to checking out (with your baby).

My room looked like

Who stayed with me

My baby spent this much time with me

My nurses

Lactation consultant visit

Pediatrician visit

Practitioner visit

How I felt physically

How I felt emotionally

My baby's feeding experiences

Other baby care experiences

Visitors

Gifts received in the hospital/birthing center

we're going home!

i t's the moment you've been waiting for. You're proud, pumped, and probably more than a little petrified. So that it doesn't become a blur in the flurry of excitement, record every detail of this special day.

I took my baby home on

The weather was

Baby wore

I wore

How I was feeling physically

How I was feeling emotionally

Who else was with me

Highlights on the way home

When I arrived at home, I

There to greet us were

Reactions of baby's sibling(s) or your pets

Other things I'd like to remember about baby's homecoming

those first postpartum days

the first week after birth will be exciting, exhilarating, and exhausting—and a blur of hectic days and sleep-deprived nights that you'll want to remember (but definitely won't unless you write it down now). Record the details here.

How I'm feeling emotionally

How I'm feeling physically

Postpartum aches and pains

My breasts feel

I'm getting this much sleep

I'm getting help from

The nicest thing my partner has done for me

The nicest things other people have done for me

The best things about not being pregnant anymore

Visitors

NOTES

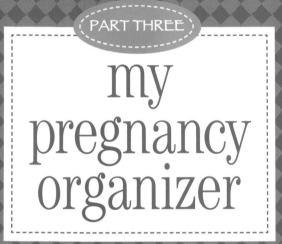

PART THREE

my
pregnancy
organizer

my pregnancy organizer

Pregnancy is full of memories and milestones you'll want to treasure forever. But it's also full of matters medical, logistical, and practical to keep track of. Thought life was hectic before? The expectant life is at least doubly so—packed with appointments that need scheduling (and remembering), doctor's orders that need following, health costs that need monitoring, layettes and furnishings that need ordering, baby names that need considering, showers that need planning, weight gain that needs watching . . . and that's just a sampling. Fortunately you don't have to try and keep it all organized in your head. That's what this Organizer section is for. To keep track of everything that needs keeping track of—from those questions you've been meaning to ask your practitioner at your next visit to the ones you'd like to ask a prospective pediatrician; from birth plans to nursery plans; from your daily calcium intake to your baby's daily movements (count those kicks, Mama!).

my prenatal care notes

Why write down every little detail of your prenatal care? So you'll never have to ask yourself, "Why didn't I write down . . . ?" So when you choose a different practitioner for your next pregnancy, you'll be able to recall the medical particulars of your first one. So when you want to compare notes on prenatal testing with your newly pregnant sister-in-law, you'll have notes to compare. So when you find yourself in a postpartum dispute with the insurance company, you'll have records to support your claim. So when you simply want to take a walk down medical memory lane, you'll be able to summon up more than just a nine-month blur.

Of course, you can't record what you don't know. Don't hesitate to ask your practitioner for the results of any test—from monthly blood pressure readings to one-time diagnostic tests of any kind. Don't hesitate, either, to tap your practitioner as a resource during or between office visits. Jot down your questions as they come up (you're sure to forget them otherwise) and your practitioner's answers as you get them (or you'll forget those, too.)

my due date

Your estimated due date will be 40 weeks from the first day of your last menstrual period and approximately 38 weeks from the date of conception. Keep in mind, though, that a full-term pregnancy can last anywhere from 38 weeks to 42 weeks, and your estimated due date is precisely that . . . estimated. Which means you can circle that magical date on your calendar, but don't use a permanent marker.

MY LAST MENSTRUAL PERIOD (LMP)   date

MY (ESTIMATED) DUE DATE   date

136

my health history

during your first prenatal visit, your practitioner will ask you lots of questions about your health; about your medical, gynecological, and obstetrical history; about lifestyle and more. To make sure you're armed with all the info you'll be asked for, do your homework before that visit (even before you've chosen a practitioner; see page 143), and bring the answers to these routine questions with you.

about your general health

Age

Prepregnancy weight   Blood type

Chronic conditions

Medications you take regularly (prescription and over the counter)

Allergies (including food allergies)

Nonobstetrical surgeries

Have you had or been vaccinated for:

   Measles

   Mumps

   Rubella

   Chicken pox

before you forget

Your first pregnancy test will probably be your home pregnancy test. Write down the results (and all the excited reactions that follow) in the Pregnancy Journal, on page 14.

137

Do you have a history of depression?

Are you currently being treated for depression? How?

Other general health issues

Primary care physician's name and phone number

NOTES

about your gynecological history

Date of your last menstrual period

Average length of your cycles

Date of last Pap smear and results

Date(s) of any abnormal Pap smears and treatment you have received

Last birth control you were using

Date you stopped using birth control

Do you have fibroids?

Do you have endometriosis?

Do you have any other gynecological conditions?

Have you ever had a sexually transmitted disease?

NOTES

about your reproductive history

Have you had any fertility issues?

Is this an IVF or other assisted-fertility pregnancy?

Number of previous pregnancies   Ages of children

Have you ever had a miscarriage? How many and when? How far along was the

pregnancy?

Have you ever had an ectopic pregnancy? When?

Have you ever had an abortion? How many?

Have you had preterm labor?   A stillbirth?

Were there any complications in your previous pregnancies?

Were there any delivery complications?

Were the deliveries vaginal or via C-section?

Did any prior delivery require the use of forceps or vacuum extraction?

Did you ever have any postpartum complications?

NOTES

about your lifestyle

Do you smoke?   How much?

Do you drink alcohol?   How much?

Do you use any recreational drugs (cocaine, marijuana)?

How much caffeinated coffee, tea, or soda do you drink?

What does your daily diet typically consist of?

Do you exercise?

If yes, what type(s) of exercise, and how often?

Do you have a cat?

Do you do a lot of gardening?

Do you take vitamins or any herbal preparations?

If yes, what kinds?

Do you use acne or wrinkle treatments?

If yes, what kind?

Are you exposed to any environmental hazards at work or at home?

What are your work conditions like? Do you stand for long periods? Do you do any

heavy lifting?

Do you work in a medical facility, in daycare, or around chemicals?

Are you under any particular emotional stress?

How is your relationship with your partner?

Have you ever been physically hurt by your partner?

NOTES

about your family history

Your birth weight   Your partner's birth weight

Your ethnicity   Your partner's ethnicity

Your partner's age

Does your partner smoke?   How much?

Does your partner drink alcohol?   How much?

Does your partner use recreational drugs?

Is your partner exposed to enviornmental hazards at work?

NOTES

Have you, your partner, or anyone in your family or your partner's family had:		
CONDITION	I OR MY FAMILY	MY PARTNER OR HIS FAMILY
Allergies, including food allergies		
Autoimmune disorder: Rheumatoid arthritis, Lupus		
Depression		
Diabetes		
Heart disease		
Hepatitis		
Hypertension		
Kidney disease		
Psychiatric disorders		
Seizure disorder		
Thyroid disease		
Autism		
Canavan disease		
Chromosomal abnormality		
Connective tissue disease		
Cystic fibrosis		
Down syndrome		
Hearing loss		
Hemophilia		
Huntington's chorea		
Mental retardation		
Muscular dystrophy		
Neural tube defects, including spina bifida, meningocele, or anencephaly		
Neurological disorders		
Phenylketonuria (PKU)		
Sickle-cell disease		
Tay-Sachs disease		
Thalassemia		
Other genetic disorders		
Difficult labor		
Preeclampsia		
Recurrent miscarriages		
Stillbirths		

choosing a practitioner

looking for the perfect partner in your pregnancy care (and who isn't)? Before you sign on, make sure you're comfortable with the practitioner you're considering by scheduling a consultation. To find out what you need to know about his or her obstetrical philosophy and style of care, and the practice setup, ask any of these questions or others you may have (you can make copies of these pages if you're planning to interview more than one practitioner). Some of the office protocol or business questions can be best answered by office personnel.

practitioner interview

Name of practitioner

Address

Phone   Fax

E-mail address

Office hours

What are your fees?

What payment options do you offer?

Do you accept my health insurance?

How long have you been in practice?

Where did you receive your training?

Affiliated hospital or birthing center

Address and phone

Affiliated lab

Address and phone

Affiliated ultrasound facility

Address and phone

What is your general philosophy about pregnancy and birth?

Who are your partners and what is the rotation schedule?

Where did they train and how long have they been with the practice?

Do I have a choice about whom I see?

Who will deliver my baby?

How many prenatal visits will I have?

How does your office handle questions that come up between visits?

How about questions that can't wait until office hours?

How do you feel about family members and friends being present at prenatal exams and during labor and birth?

What is your definition of a high-risk pregnancy?

What percentage of women in your practice have C-sections?

Are you open to my hiring a doula?

How do you feel about written birth plans?

At what point in labor will you try to be with me?

What tests do you recommend/perform:

☐ CVS   ☐ GLUCOSE SCREENING

☐ AMNIOCENTESIS   ☐ GROUP B STREP

☐ COMBINED SCREENING   ☐ NONSTRESS TEST

☐ INTEGRATED SCREENING   ☐ BIOPHYSICAL PROFILE

☐ TRIPLE/QUAD SCREEN   ☐

☐ EARLY ULTRASOUND   ☐

☐ LEVEL II ULTRASOUND

What is your policy on:

Scheduled C-sections

Inducing labor

Continuous IV during labor

Fetal monitoring during labor

Pain medications during labor

Unmedicated birth

Episiotomy

Forceps and vacuum extraction

Labor augmentation

Artificial rupture of membranes

VBAC (vaginal birth after previous C-section)

Breastfeeding immediately after birth

Home birth

Water birth

Complementary and alternative therapies

Additional questions specific to a midwife:

What is your midwifery training?

What certifications do you have?

Will you attend my home birth?

Will you attend my water birth?

What protocols do you have in place if I or my baby need emergency treatment?

Do you have obstetrical backup?

Who is your backup doctor?

Will I meet your medical backup?

If I'm planning a home or birthing-center delivery, under what circumstances would you require that I be transferred to a hospital?

NOTES

practitioner's recommendations

Over the course of your pregnancy, you'll be getting plenty of advice from your practitioner—recommendations on everything from which exercises get the green light to which medications get the red light, from how much weight you should aim to gain to how much coffee you can drink, from how long you can keep traveling to what you should do if you start spotting. Jot down all those recommendations here so you won't forget them.

Optimal total weight gain

Suggested rate of gain

Prescription medications I can safely take

Over-the-counter medications I can safely take

Over-the-counter medications that I shouldn't take

Prenatal vitamin

Other supplements (such as iron, calcium, herbal)

Dietary guidelines

Food and drinks that are off-limits

Guidelines for:

Complementary and alternative therapies

Exercise

Sex/orgasm

Work

Travel

Skin and hair products/treatments that are off-limits

Limitations on activities, if any

Recommendations for:

Abdominal aches

Aversions

Backache

Bleeding gums

Bloating

Breast tenderness

Carpal tunnel syndrome

Constipation

Cravings

Fatigue

Headaches

Heartburn

Hemorrhoids

Leg cramps

Morning sickness

Sciatica

Swelling

Varicose veins

Call immediately if experiencing

Call the same day if experiencing

Call when contractions are this far apart

Other recommendations or instructions

NOTES

prenatal tests

Can't wait to get to know your baby? Though you won't be meeting face to adorable face for months to come, you'll be getting to know lots about your baby through prenatal tests. From blood tests to ultrasounds to amniocentesis, you're sure to have at least one or two prenatal screenings and diagnostic tests while you're expecting (and probably many more). Use these pages to record all the results.

first-trimester screening and diagnostic tests

Maternal/Combined Serum Screening

Date/Place

When/where to call for results

Practitioner

Results

Follow-up tests needed, if any

Follow-up results

Ultrasound

Date/Place

When/where to call for results

Practitioner

Results

Follow-up tests needed, if any

Follow-up results

Chorionic Villus Sampling

Date/Place

When/where to call for results

Practitioner

Results

Follow-up tests needed, if any

Follow-up results

second-trimester screening and diagnostic tests

Integrated Screening

Date/Place

When/where to call for results

Practitioner

Results

Follow-up tests needed, if any

Follow-up results

Triple (or Quad) Screen

Date/Place

When/where to call for results

Practitioner

Results

Follow-up tests needed, if any

Follow-up results

Amniocentesis

Date/Place

When/where to call for results

Practitioner

Results

Follow-up tests needed, if any

Follow-up results

Ultrasound

Date/Place

When/where to call for results

Practitioner

Results

Follow-up tests needed, if any

Follow-up results

Ultrasound

Date/Place

When/where to call for results

Practitioner

Results

Follow-up tests needed, if any

Follow-up results

Ultrasound

Date/Place

When/where to call for results

Practitioner

Results

Follow-up tests needed, if any

Follow-up results

NOTES

before you forget

Remember to record your reaction and that of your partner to your ultrasounds in the journal section of this organizer (pages 15 and 47). There's also a place to paste ultrasound photos there.

Nonstress Test

Date/Place

When/where to call for results

Practitioner

Results

Follow-up tests needed, if any

Follow-up results

Biophysical Profile

Date/Place

When/where to call for results

Practitioner

Results

Follow-up tests needed, if any

Follow-up results

Contraction-Stress Test

Date/Place

When/where to call for results

Practitioner

Results

Follow-up tests needed, if any

Follow-up results

Other Screenings and Diagnostic Tests, Dates and Results

Allergies, including food allergies

Glucose screening test

Glucose tolerance test

Group B strep

hCG levels

Hematocrit or hemoglobin

Hepatitis B

HIV

Pap smear

RH status

Rubella titer

Tests for STDs

Toxoplasmosis test

Genetic tests (Tay-Sachs, sickle-cell anemia, etc.)

Other

practitioner visits

U sed to going to the doctor once a year? Get ready to step up that schedule—a lot. Now that you're expecting, expect to visit your practitioner for prenatal care at least once a month—and as you get closer to D-day, every week or so. All your visits will be information-packed, so to make sure you walk away with that information; jot it down on these pages.

practitioner's visit

Practitioner seen   Date/Time

Weight   Blood pressure   Pulse

Pregnancy blood/urine test results

hCG levels

Urinalysis: Sugar   Protein

Other tests

Fetal heart rate (if seen)

Questions to ask at this visit

1

Answer

2

Answer

3

Answer

Practitioner's instructions and recommendations

between visits

Calls made to practitioner

Date called

Reason

Instructions/Advice

Date called

Reason

Instructions/Advice

Date called

Reason

Instructions/Advice

Things to remember for the next visit

practitioner's visit

Practitioner seen   Date/Time

Weight   Blood pressure   Pulse

hGC levels

Urinalysis: Sugar   Protein

Other tests

Fetal heart rate

Questions to ask at this visit

1

Answer

2

Answer

3

Answer

4

Answer

5

Answer

before you forget

Remember to record
your reaction and that
of your partner to
hearing your baby's
heartbeat in the
journal section of this
organizer (page 24).

158

Practitioner's instructions and recommendations

between visits

Calls made to practitioner

Date called

Reason

Instructions/Advice

Date called

Reason

Instructions/Advice

Date called

Reason

Instructions/Advice

Things to remember for the next visit

practitioner's visit

Practitioner seen .... Date/Time ....

Weight .... Blood pressure .... Pulse ....

Urinalysis: Sugar .... Protein ....

Other tests ....

....

Height of fundus .... Fetal heart rate ....

Questions to ask at this visit

1 ....

Answer ....

....

2 ....

Answer ....

....

3 ....

Answer ....

....

4 ....

Answer ....

....

5 ....

Answer ....

....

6 ....

Answer ....

Practitioner's instructions and recommendations

_____

_____

_____

_____

between visits

Calls made to practitioner

Date called _____

Reason _____

_____

Instructions/Advice _____

Date called _____

Reason _____

_____

Instructions/Advice _____

Date called _____

Reason _____

_____

Instructions/Advice _____

Things to remember for the next visit

_____

_____

_____

practitioner's visit

Practitioner seen   Date/Time

Weight   Blood pressure   Pulse

Urinalysis: Sugar   Protein

Other tests

Height of fundus   Fetal heart rate

Questions to ask at this visit

1

Answer

2

Answer

3

Answer

4

Answer

5

Answer

6

Answer

Practitioner's instructions and recommendations

_____
_____
_____
_____

between visits

Calls made to practitioner

Date called

Reason

Instructions/Advice

Date called

Reason

Instructions/Advice

Date called

Reason

Instructions/Advice

Things to remember for the next visit

_____
_____

practitioner's visit

Practitioner seen   Date/Time

Weight   Blood pressure   Pulse

Urinalysis: Sugar   Protein

Other tests

Height of fundus   Fetal heart rate

Questions to ask at this visit

1

Answer

2

Answer

3

Answer

4

Answer

5

Answer

6

Answer

Practitioner's instructions and recommendations

between visits

Calls made to practitioner

Date called

Reason

Instructions/Advice

Date called

Reason

Instructions/Advice

Date called

Reason

Instructions/Advice

Things to remember for the next visit

practitioner's visit

Practitioner seen   Date/Time

Weight   Blood pressure   Pulse

Urinalysis: Sugar   Protein

Other tests

Height of fundus   Fetal heart rate

Questions to ask at this visit

1

Answer

2

Answer

3

Answer

4

Answer

5

Answer

6

Answer

Practitioner's instructions and recommendations

between visits

Calls made to practitioner

Date called

Reason

Instructions/Advice

Date called

Reason

Instructions/Advice

Date called

Reason

Instructions/Advice

Things to remember for the next visit

practitioner's visit

Practitioner seen   Date/Time

Weight   Blood pressure   Pulse

Urinalysis: Sugar   Protein

Other tests

Height of fundus   Fetal heart rate

Questions to ask at this visit

1

Answer

2

Answer

3

Answer

4

Answer

5

Answer

6

Answer

Practitioner's instructions and recommendations

between visits

Calls made to practitioner

Date called

Reason

Instructions/Advice

Date called

Reason

Instructions/Advice

Date called

Reason

Instructions/Advice

Things to remember for the next visit

practitioner's visit

Practitioner seen   Date/Time

Weight   Blood pressure   Pulse

Urinalysis: Sugar   Protein

Other tests

Height of fundus   Fetal heart rate

Questions to ask at this visit

1

Answer

2

Answer

3

Answer

4

Answer

5

Answer

6

Answer

Practitioner's instructions and recommendations

between visits

Calls made to practitioner

Date called

Reason

Instructions/Advice

Date called

Reason

Instructions/Advice

Date called

Reason

Instructions/Advice

Things to remember for the next visit

practitioner's visit

Practitioner seen   Date/Time

Weight   Blood pressure   Pulse

Urinalysis: Sugar   Protein

Other tests

Height of fundus   Fetal heart rate

Dilation   Effacement   Station

Questions to ask at this visit

1

Answer

2

Answer

3

Answer

4

Answer

5

Answer

Practitioner's instructions and recommendations

_____

_____

_____

_____

between visits

Calls made to practitioner

Date called _____

Reason _____

_____

Instructions/Advice _____

Date called _____

Reason _____

_____

Instructions/Advice _____

Date called _____

Reason _____

_____

Instructions/Advice _____

Things to remember for the next visit

_____

_____

_____

practitioner's visit

Practitioner seen   Date/Time

Weight   Blood pressure   Pulse

Urinalysis: Sugar   Protein

Other tests

Height of fundus   Fetal heart rate

Dilation   Effacement   Station

Questions to ask at this visit

1

Answer

2

Answer

3

Answer

4

Answer

5

Answer

Practitioner's instructions and recommendations

_____

_____

_____

_____

between visits

Calls made to practitioner

Date called

Reason

_____

Instructions/Advice

_____

Date called

Reason

_____

Instructions/Advice

_____

Date called

Reason

_____

Instructions/Advice

_____

Things to remember for the next visit

_____

_____

practitioner's visit

Practitioner seen .... Date/Time ....

Weight .... Blood pressure .... Pulse ....

Urinalysis: Sugar .... Protein ....

Other tests ....

Height of fundus .... Fetal heart rate ....

Dilation .... Effacement .... Station ....

Questions to ask at this visit

1 ....

Answer ....

2 ....

Answer ....

3 ....

Answer ....

4 ....

Answer ....

5 ....

Answer ....

Practitioner's instructions and recommendations

between visits

Calls made to practitioner

Date called

Reason

Instructions/Advice

Date called

Reason

Instructions/Advice

Date called

Reason

Instructions/Advice

Things to remember for the next visit

practitioner's visit

Practitioner seen   Date/Time

Weight   Blood pressure   Pulse

Urinalysis: Sugar   Protein

Other tests

Height of fundus   Fetal heart rate

Dilation   Effacement   Station

Questions to ask at this visit

1

Answer

2

Answer

3

Answer

4

Answer

5

Answer

Practitioner's instructions and recommendations

between visits

Calls made to practitioner

Date called

Reason

Instructions/Advice

Date called

Reason

Instructions/Advice

Date called

Reason

Instructions/Advice

Things to remember for the next visit

practitioner's visit

Practitioner seen   Date/Time

Weight   Blood pressure   Pulse

Urinalysis: Sugar   Protein

Other tests

Height of fundus   Fetal heart rate

Dilation   Effacement   Station

Questions to ask at this visit

1

Answer

2

Answer

3

Answer

4

Answer

5

Answer

Practitioner's instructions and recommendations

between visits

Calls made to practitioner

Date called

Reason

Instructions/Advice

Date called

Reason

Instructions/Advice

Date called

Reason

Instructions/Advice

Things to remember for the next visit

pregnancy
medical finances

b abies cost a lot of money—even before they're born. So that you don't get lost under a sea of bills and insurance papers, use these pages to record all your medical financial information.

Insurance company/HMO

Address

Phone

Policyholder's name and ID no.

Co-pay

My practitioner accepts these methods of payment

I have chosen this payment schedule

Notes

Pregnancy-Related Services

Service   Date

Provider

Address

Phone   Fax

Financial arrangement/fee

How paid   Date paid

Amount reimbursed

NOTES

Service   Date

Provider

Address

Phone   Fax

Financial arrangement/fee

How paid   Date paid

Amount reimbursed

NOTES

Service   Date

Provider

Address

Phone   Fax

Financial arrangement/fee

How paid   Date paid

Amount reimbursed

NOTES

Service _____ Date _____

Provider _____

Address _____

_____

Phone _____ Fax _____

Financial arrangement/fee _____

How paid _____ Date paid _____

Amount reimbursed _____

NOTES _____

Service _____ Date _____

Provider _____

Address _____

_____

Phone _____ Fax _____

Financial arrangement/fee _____

How paid _____ Date paid _____

Amount reimbursed _____

NOTES _____

Service _____ Date _____

Provider _____

Address _____

_____

Phone _____ Fax _____

Financial arrangement/fee

How paid _____ Date paid _____

Amount reimbursed _____

NOTES _____

Service _____ Date _____

Provider _____

Address _____

Phone _____ Fax _____

Financial arrangement/fee _____

How paid _____ Date paid _____

Amount reimbursed _____

NOTES _____

Service _____ Date _____

Provider _____

Address _____

Phone _____ Fax _____

Financial arrangement/fee _____

How paid _____ Date paid _____

Amount reimbursed _____

NOTES _____

pregnancy trackers

a re you the kind of person who needs to keep track of absolutely everything in order to get it all done? Then this is your kind of section. Here you'll find a place to keep track of your exercise program (whether you're shooting for once a week or twice a day), your Pregnancy Diet (so you don't forget what you had for breakfast by the time the lunch cart rolls into the conference room), your weight-gain progress (though this may be something you'd rather forget), and your baby's movements (once you're counting, which won't be until 28 weeks). Input into your trackers as often— or as infrequently—as you like. You may find, for instance, that filling out your food tracker once a week is enough—or that writing down your weight once a month is more than enough.

exercise tracker

e xercising for two doesn't mean exercising twice as hard or twice as often. You will get the best benefits if you exercise consistently while you're expecting. Whether your exercise goal will be met by two fifteen-minute walks a day, a three-mile power walk three times a week, or by mixing it up to suit your mood (a yoga class twice a week, a swim once a week, an evening stroll whenever you have the energy), keeping track will help you stay on track (or on the track). It'll also help motivate you—writing down your accomplishments always does!

WEEK:	TYPE OF EXERCISE	DURATION	HOW I FELT AFTERWARD
Sunday			
Monday			
Tuesday			
Wednesday			
Thursday			
Friday			
Saturday			

WEEK:	TYPE OF EXERCISE	DURATION	HOW I FELT AFTERWARD
Sunday			
Monday			
Tuesday			
Wednesday			
Thursday			
Friday			
Saturday			

WEEK:	TYPE OF EXERCISE	DURATION	HOW I FELT AFTERWARD
Sunday			
Monday			
Tuesday			
Wednesday			
Thursday			
Friday			
Saturday			

WEEK:	TYPE OF EXERCISE	DURATION	HOW I FELT AFTERWARD
Sunday			
Monday			
Tuesday			
Wednesday			
Thursday			
Friday			
Saturday			

WEEK:	TYPE OF EXERCISE	DURATION	HOW I FELT AFTERWARD
Sunday			
Monday			
Tuesday			
Wednesday			
Thursday			
Friday			
Saturday			

WEEK:	TYPE OF EXERCISE	DURATION	HOW I FELT AFTERWARD
Sunday			
Monday			
Tuesday			
Wednesday			
Thursday			
Friday			
Saturday			

WEEK:	TYPE OF EXERCISE	DURATION	HOW I FELT AFTERWARD
Sunday			
Monday			
Tuesday			
Wednesday			
Thursday			
Friday			
Saturday			

WEEK:	TYPE OF EXERCISE	DURATION	HOW I FELT AFTERWARD
Sunday			
Monday			
Tuesday			
Wednesday			
Thursday			
Friday			
Saturday			

WEEK:	TYPE OF EXERCISE	DURATION	HOW I FELT AFTERWARD
Sunday			
Monday			
Tuesday			
Wednesday			
Thursday			
Friday			
Saturday			

WEEK:	TYPE OF EXERCISE	DURATION	HOW I FELT AFTERWARD
Sunday			
Monday			
Tuesday			
Wednesday			
Thursday			
Friday			
Saturday			

WEEK:	TYPE OF EXERCISE	DURATION	HOW I FELT AFTERWARD
Sunday			
Monday			
Tuesday			
Wednesday			
Thursday			
Friday			
Saturday			

WEEK:	TYPE OF EXERCISE	DURATION	HOW I FELT AFTERWARD
Sunday			
Monday			
Tuesday			
Wednesday			
Thursday			
Friday			
Saturday			

WEEK:	TYPE OF EXERCISE	DURATION	HOW I FELT AFTERWARD
Sunday			
Monday			
Tuesday			
Wednesday			
Thursday			
Friday			
Saturday			

WEEK:	TYPE OF EXERCISE	DURATION	HOW I FELT AFTERWARD
Sunday			
Monday			
Tuesday			
Wednesday			
Thursday			
Friday			
Saturday			

WEEK:	TYPE OF EXERCISE	DURATION	HOW I FELT AFTERWARD
Sunday			
Monday			
Tuesday			
Wednesday			
Thursday			
Friday			
Saturday			

WEEK:	TYPE OF EXERCISE	DURATION	HOW I FELT AFTERWARD
Sunday			
Monday			
Tuesday			
Wednesday			
Thursday			
Friday			
Saturday			

WEEK:	TYPE OF EXERCISE	DURATION	HOW I FELT AFTERWARD
Sunday			
Monday			
Tuesday			
Wednesday			
Thursday			
Friday			
Saturday			

WEEK:	TYPE OF EXERCISE	DURATION	HOW I FELT AFTERWARD
Sunday			
Monday			
Tuesday			
Wednesday			
Thursday			
Friday			
Saturday			

WEEK:	TYPE OF EXERCISE	DURATION	HOW I FELT AFTERWARD
Sunday			
Monday			
Tuesday			
Wednesday			
Thursday			
Friday			
Saturday			

WEEK:	TYPE OF EXERCISE	DURATION	HOW I FELT AFTERWARD
Sunday			
Monday			
Tuesday			
Wednesday			
Thursday			
Friday			
Saturday			

WEEK:	TYPE OF EXERCISE	DURATION	HOW I FELT AFTERWARD
Sunday			
Monday			
Tuesday			
Wednesday			
Thursday			
Friday			
Saturday			

WEEK:	TYPE OF EXERCISE	DURATION	HOW I FELT AFTERWARD
Sunday			
Monday			
Tuesday			
Wednesday			
Thursday			
Friday			
Saturday			

WEEK:	TYPE OF EXERCISE	DURATION	HOW I FELT AFTERWARD
Sunday			
Monday			
Tuesday			
Wednesday			
Thursday			
Friday			
Saturday			

WEEK:	TYPE OF EXERCISE	DURATION	HOW I FELT AFTERWARD
Sunday			
Monday			
Tuesday			
Wednesday			
Thursday			
Friday			
Saturday			

WEEK:	TYPE OF EXERCISE	DURATION	HOW I FELT AFTERWARD
Sunday			
Monday			
Tuesday			
Wednesday			
Thursday			
Friday			
Saturday			

WEEK:	TYPE OF EXERCISE	DURATION	HOW I FELT AFTERWARD
Sunday			
Monday			
Tuesday			
Wednesday			
Thursday			
Friday			
Saturday			

WEEK:	TYPE OF EXERCISE	DURATION	HOW I FELT AFTERWARD
Sunday			
Monday			
Tuesday			
Wednesday			
Thursday			
Friday			
Saturday			

WEEK:	TYPE OF EXERCISE	DURATION	HOW I FELT AFTERWARD
Sunday			
Monday			
Tuesday			
Wednesday			
Thursday			
Friday			
Saturday			

WEEK:	TYPE OF EXERCISE	DURATION	HOW I FELT AFTERWARD
Sunday			
Monday			
Tuesday			
Wednesday			
Thursday			
Friday			
Saturday			

WEEK:	TYPE OF EXERCISE	DURATION	HOW I FELT AFTERWARD
Sunday			
Monday			
Tuesday			
Wednesday			
Thursday			
Friday			
Saturday			

WEEK:	TYPE OF EXERCISE	DURATION	HOW I FELT AFTERWARD
Sunday			
Monday			
Tuesday			
Wednesday			
Thursday			
Friday			
Saturday			

WEEK:	TYPE OF EXERCISE	DURATION	HOW I FELT AFTERWARD
Sunday			
Monday			
Tuesday			
Wednesday			
Thursday			
Friday			
Saturday			

WEEK:	TYPE OF EXERCISE	DURATION	HOW I FELT AFTERWARD
Sunday			
Monday			
Tuesday			
Wednesday			
Thursday			
Friday			
Saturday			

WEEK:	TYPE OF EXERCISE	DURATION	HOW I FELT AFTERWARD
Sunday			
Monday			
Tuesday			
Wednesday			
Thursday			
Friday			
Saturday			

WEEK:	TYPE OF EXERCISE	DURATION	HOW I FELT AFTERWARD
Sunday			
Monday			
Tuesday			
Wednesday			
Thursday			
Friday			
Saturday			

WEEK:	TYPE OF EXERCISE	DURATION	HOW I FELT AFTERWARD
Sunday			
Monday			
Tuesday			
Wednesday			
Thursday			
Friday			
Saturday			

diet tracker

luckily, eating well when you're expecting isn't all that different from eating well at any other time. The Pregnancy Diet—an eating plan designed to give your baby the best possible start in life—divides the nutrients and calories you need into twelve convenient categories (aka The Daily Dozen), of which you should aim to get a certain number of servings daily. Many foods count toward more than one category (for example, Calcium foods often fill a Protein requirement), allowing you to double (or triple) up on nutrients while keeping your caloric intake in check. You can keep track of your Daily Dozen on these pages—though, actually, you'll only have to keep track of 11 of them. Calories aren't listed here because you don't need to count them (just keep your eye on the scale to determine whether you're getting too many, too few, or just the right number). (For more on what they are, see *What to Expect When You're Expecting* or *What to Expect: Eating Well When You're Expecting.* For sample daily menus to help you reach your Daily Dozen deliciously, go to whattoexpect.com.)

daily dozen diary

WEEK:	S	M	T	W	T	F	S
Protein foods (3)							
Calcium foods (4)							
Vitamin C foods (3)							
Green leafy/Yellows (3 to 4)							
Other fruits & vegetables (1 to 2)							
Whole grains & legumes (6 or more)							
Iron-rich foods (some daily)							
Fat (4)							
Salt							
Fluids (at least 8)							
Prenatal vitamin							

daily dozen diary

WEEK:	S	M	T	W	T	F	S
Protein foods (3)							
Calcium foods (4)							
Vitamin C foods (3)							
Green leafy/Yellows (3 to 4)							
Other fruits & vegetables (1 to 2)							
Whole grains & legumes (6 or more)							
Iron-rich foods (some daily)							
Fat (4)							
Salt							
Fluids (at least 8)							
Prenatal vitamin							

daily dozen diary

WEEK:	S	M	T	W	T	F	S
Protein foods (3)							
Calcium foods (4)							
Vitamin C foods (3)							
Green leafy/Yellows (3 to 4)							
Other fruits & vegetables (1 to 2)							
Whole grains & legumes (6 or more)							
Iron-rich foods (some daily)							
Fat (4)							
Salt							
Fluids (at least 8)							
Prenatal vitamin							

daily dozen diary

WEEK:	S	M	T	W	T	F	S
Protein foods (3)							
Calcium foods (4)							
Vitamin C foods (3)							
Green leafy/Yellows (3 to 4)							
Other fruits & vegetables (1 to 2)							
Whole grains & legumes (6 or more)							
Iron-rich foods (some daily)							
Fat (4)							
Salt							
Fluids (at least 8)							
Prenatal vitamin							

daily dozen diary

WEEK:	S	M	T	W	T	F	S
Protein foods (3)							
Calcium foods (4)							
Vitamin C foods (3)							
Green leafy/Yellows (3 to 4)							
Other fruits & vegetables (1 to 2)							
Whole grains & legumes (6 or more)							
Iron-rich foods (some daily)							
Fat (4)							
Salt							
Fluids (at least 8)							
Prenatal vitamin							

daily dozen diary

WEEK:	S	M	T	W	T	F	S
Protein foods (3)							
Calcium foods (4)							
Vitamin C foods (3)							
Green leafy/Yellows (3 to 4)							
Other fruits & vegetables (1 to 2)							
Whole grains & legumes (6 or more)							
Iron-rich foods (some daily)							
Fat (4)							
Salt							
Fluids (at least 8)							
Prenatal vitamin							

daily dozen diary

WEEK:	S	M	T	W	T	F	S
Protein foods (3)							
Calcium foods (4)							
Vitamin C foods (3)							
Green leafy/Yellows (3 to 4)							
Other fruits & vegetables (1 to 2)							
Whole grains & legumes (6 or more)							
Iron-rich foods (some daily)							
Fat (4)							
Salt							
Fluids (at least 8)							
Prenatal vitamin							

daily dozen diary

WEEK:	S	M	T	W	T	F	S
Protein foods (3)							
Calcium foods (4)							
Vitamin C foods (3)							
Green leafy/Yellows (3 to 4)							
Other fruits & vegetables (1 to 2)							
Whole grains & legumes (6 or more)							
Iron-rich foods (some daily)							
Fat (4)							
Salt							
Fluids (at least 8)							
Prenatal vitamin							

daily dozen diary

WEEK:	S	M	T	W	T	F	S
Protein foods (3)							
Calcium foods (4)							
Vitamin C foods (3)							
Green leafy/Yellows (3 to 4)							
Other fruits & vegetables (1 to 2)							
Whole grains & legumes (6 or more)							
Iron-rich foods (some daily)							
Fat (4)							
Salt							
Fluids (at least 8)							
Prenatal vitamin							

daily dozen diary

WEEK:	S	M	T	W	T	F	S
Protein foods (3)							
Calcium foods (4)							
Vitamin C foods (3)							
Green leafy/Yellows (3 to 4)							
Other fruits & vegetables (1 to 2)							
Whole grains & legumes (6 or more)							
Iron-rich foods (some daily)							
Fat (4)							
Salt							
Fluids (at least 8)							
Prenatal vitamin							

daily dozen diary

WEEK:	S	M	T	W	T	F	S
Protein foods (3)							
Calcium foods (4)							
Vitamin C foods (3)							
Green leafy/Yellows (3 to 4)							
Other fruits & vegetables (1 to 2)							
Whole grains & legumes (6 or more)							
Iron-rich foods (some daily)							
Fat (4)							
Salt							
Fluids (at least 8)							
Prenatal vitamin							

daily dozen diary

WEEK:	S	M	T	W	T	F	S
Protein foods (3)							
Calcium foods (4)							
Vitamin C foods (3)							
Green leafy/Yellows (3 to 4)							
Other fruits & vegetables (1 to 2)							
Whole grains & legumes (6 or more)							
Iron-rich foods (some daily)							
Fat (4)							
Salt							
Fluids (at least 8)							
Prenatal vitamin							

daily dozen diary

WEEK:	S	M	T	W	T	F	S
Protein foods (3)							
Calcium foods (4)							
Vitamin C foods (3)							
Green leafy/Yellows (3 to 4)							
Other fruits & vegetables (1 to 2)							
Whole grains & legumes (6 or more)							
Iron-rich foods (some daily)							
Fat (4)							
Salt							
Fluids (at least 8)							
Prenatal vitamin							

daily dozen diary

WEEK:	S	M	T	W	T	F	S
Protein foods (3)							
Calcium foods (4)							
Vitamin C foods (3)							
Green leafy/Yellows (3 to 4)							
Other fruits & vegetables (1 to 2)							
Whole grains & legumes (6 or more)							
Iron-rich foods (some daily)							
Fat (4)							
Salt							
Fluids (at least 8)							
Prenatal vitamin							

daily dozen diary

WEEK:	S	M	T	W	T	F	S
Protein foods (3)							
Calcium foods (4)							
Vitamin C foods (3)							
Green leafy/Yellows (3 to 4)							
Other fruits & v egetables (1 to 2)							
Whole grains & legumes (6 or more)							
Iron-rich foods (some daily)							
Fat (4)							
Salt							
Fluids (at least 8)							
Prenatal vitamin							

daily dozen diary

WEEK:	S	M	T	W	T	F	S
Protein foods (3)							
Calcium foods (4)							
Vitamin C foods (3)							
Green leafy/Yellows (3 to 4)							
Other fruits & vegetables (1 to 2)							
Whole grains & legumes (6 or more)							
Iron-rich foods (some daily)							
Fat (4)							
Salt							
Fluids (at least 8)							
Prenatal vitamin							

daily dozen diary

WEEK:	S	M	T	W	T	F	S
Protein foods (3)							
Calcium foods (4)							
Vitamin C foods (3)							
Green leafy/Yellows (3 to 4)							
Other fruits & vegetables (1 to 2)							
Whole grains & legumes (6 or more)							
Iron-rich foods (some daily)							
Fat (4)							
Salt							
Fluids (at least 8)							
Prenatal vitamin							

daily dozen diary

WEEK:	S	M	T	W	T	F	S
Protein foods (3)							
Calcium foods (4)							
Vitamin C foods (3)							
Green leafy/Yellows (3 to 4)							
Other fruits & vegetables (1 to 2)							
Whole grains & legumes (6 or more)							
Iron-rich foods (some daily)							
Fat (4)							
Salt							
Fluids (at least 8)							
Prenatal vitamin							

daily dozen diary

WEEK:	S	M	T	W	T	F	S
Protein foods (3)							
Calcium foods (4)							
Vitamin C foods (3)							
Green leafy/Yellows (3 to 4)							
Other fruits & vegetables (1 to 2)							
Whole grains & legumes (6 or more)							
Iron-rich foods (some daily)							
Fat (4)							
Salt							
Fluids (at least 8)							
Prenatal vitamin							

daily dozen diary

WEEK:	S	M	T	W	T	F	S
Protein foods (3)							
Calcium foods (4)							
Vitamin C foods (3)							
Green leafy/Yellows (3 to 4)							
Other fruits & vegetables (1 to 2)							
Whole grains & legumes (6 or more)							
Iron-rich foods (some daily)							
Fat (4)							
Salt							
Fluids (at least 8)							
Prenatal vitamin							

daily dozen diary

WEEK:	S	M	T	W	T	F	S
Protein foods (3)							
Calcium foods (4)							
Vitamin C foods (3)							
Green leafy/Yellows (3 to 4)							
Other fruits & vegetables (1 to 2)							
Whole grains & legumes (6 or more)							
Iron-rich foods (some daily)							
Fat (4)							
Salt							
Fluids (at least 8)							
Prenatal vitamin							

daily dozen diary

WEEK:	S	M	T	W	T	F	S
Protein foods (3)							
Calcium foods (4)							
Vitamin C foods (3)							
Green leafy/Yellows (3 to 4)							
Other fruits & vegetables (1 to 2)							
Whole grains & legumes (6 or more)							
Iron-rich foods (some daily)							
Fat (4)							
Salt							
Fluids (at least 8)							
Prenatal vitamin							

daily dozen diary

WEEK:	S	M	T	W	T	F	S
Protein foods (3)							
Calcium foods (4)							
Vitamin C foods (3)							
Green leafy/Yellows (3 to 4)							
Other fruits & vegetables (1 to 2)							
Whole grains & legumes (6 or more)							
Iron-rich foods (some daily)							
Fat (4)							
Salt							
Fluids (at least 8)							
Prenatal vitamin							

daily dozen diary

WEEK:	S	M	T	W	T	F	S
Protein foods (3)							
Calcium foods (4)							
Vitamin C foods (3)							
Green leafy/Yellows (3 to 4)							
Other fruits & vegetables (1 to 2)							
Whole grains & legumes (6 or more)							
Iron-rich foods (some daily)							
Fat (4)							
Salt							
Fluids (at least 8)							
Prenatal vitamin							

daily dozen diary

WEEK:	S	M	T	W	T	F	S
Protein foods (3)							
Calcium foods (4)							
Vitamin C foods (3)							
Green leafy/Yellows (3 to 4)							
Other fruits & vegetables (1 to 2)							
Whole grains & legumes (6 or more)							
Iron-rich foods (some daily)							
Fat (4)							
Salt							
Fluids (at least 8)							
Prenatal vitamin							

daily dozen diary

WEEK:	S	M	T	W	T	F	S
Protein foods (3)							
Calcium foods (4)							
Vitamin C foods (3)							
Green leafy/Yellows (3 to 4)							
Other fruits & vegetables (1 to 2)							
Whole grains & legumes (6 or more)							
Iron-rich foods (some daily)							
Fat (4)							
Salt							
Fluids (at least 8)							
Prenatal vitamin							

daily dozen diary

WEEK:	S	M	T	W	T	F	S
Protein foods (3)							
Calcium foods (4)							
Vitamin C foods (3)							
Green leafy/Yellows (3 to 4)							
Other fruits & vegetables (1 to 2)							
Whole grains & legumes (6 or more)							
Iron-rich foods (some daily)							
Fat (4)							
Salt							
Fluids (at least 8)							
Prenatal vitamin							

daily dozen diary

WEEK:	S	M	T	W	T	F	S
Protein foods (3)							
Calcium foods (4)							
Vitamin C foods (3)							
Green leafy/Yellows (3 to 4)							
Other fruits & vegetables (1 to 2)							
Whole grains & legumes (6 or more)							
Iron-rich foods (some daily)							
Fat (4)							
Salt							
Fluids (at least 8)							
Prenatal vitamin							

daily dozen diary

WEEK:	S	M	T	W	T	F	S
Protein foods (3)							
Calcium foods (4)							
Vitamin C foods (3)							
Green leafy/Yellows (3 to 4)							
Other fruits & vegetables (1 to 2)							
Whole grains & legumes (6 or more)							
Iron-rich foods (some daily)							
Fat (4)							
Salt							
Fluids (at least 8)							
Prenatal vitamin							

daily dozen diary

WEEK:	S	M	T	W	T	F	S
Protein foods (3)							
Calcium foods (4)							
Vitamin C foods (3)							
Green leafy/Yellows (3 to 4)							
Other fruits & vegetables (1 to 2)							
Whole grains & legumes (6 or more)							
Iron-rich foods (some daily)							
Fat (4)							
Salt							
Fluids (at least 8)							
Prenatal vitamin							

daily dozen diary

WEEK:	S	M	T	W	T	F	S
Protein foods (3)							
Calcium foods (4)							
Vitamin C foods (3)							
Green leafy/Yellows (3 to 4)							
Other fruits & vegetables (1 to 2)							
Whole grains & legumes (6 or more)							
Iron-rich foods (some daily)							
Fat (4)							
Salt							
Fluids (at least 8)							
Prenatal vitamin							

daily dozen diary

WEEK:	S	M	T	W	T	F	S
Protein foods (3)							
Calcium foods (4)							
Vitamin C foods (3)							
Green leafy/Yellows (3 to 4)							
Other fruits & vegetables (1 to 2)							
Whole grains & legumes (6 or more)							
Iron-rich foods (some daily)							
Fat (4)							
Salt							
Fluids (at least 8)							
Prenatal vitamin							

daily dozen diary

WEEK:	S	M	T	W	T	F	S
Protein foods (3)							
Calcium foods (4)							
Vitamin C foods (3)							
Green leafy/Yellows (3 to 4)							
Other fruits & vegetables (1 to 2)							
Whole grains & legumes (6 or more)							
Iron-rich foods (some daily)							
Fat (4)							
Salt							
Fluids (at least 8)							
Prenatal vitamin							

daily dozen diary

WEEK:	S	M	T	W	T	F	S
Protein foods (3)							
Calcium foods (4)							
Vitamin C foods (3)							
Green leafy/Yellows (3 to 4)							
Other fruits & vegetables (1 to 2)							
Whole grains & legumes (6 or more)							
Iron-rich foods (some daily)							
Fat (4)							
Salt							
Fluids (at least 8)							
Prenatal vitamin							

daily dozen diary

WEEK:	S	M	T	W	T	F	S
Protein foods (3)							
Calcium foods (4)							
Vitamin C foods (3)							
Green leafy/Yellows (3 to 4)							
Other fruits & vegetables (1 to 2)							
Whole grains & legumes (6 or more)							
Iron-rich foods (some daily)							
Fat (4)							
Salt							
Fluids (at least 8)							
Prenatal vitamin							

daily dozen diary

WEEK:	S	M	T	W	T	F	S
Protein foods (3)							
Calcium foods (4)							
Vitamin C foods (3)							
Green leafy/Yellows (3 to 4)							
Other fruits & vegetables (1 to 2)							
Whole grains & legumes (6 or more)							
Iron-rich foods (some daily)							
Fat (4)							
Salt							
Fluids (at least 8)							
Prenatal vitamin							

daily dozen diary

WEEK:	S	M	T	W	T	F	S
Protein foods (3)							
Calcium foods (4)							
Vitamin C foods (3)							
Green leafy/Yellows (3 to 4)							
Other fruits & vegetables (1 to 2)							
Whole grains & legumes (6 or more)							
Iron-rich foods (some daily)							
Fat (4)							
Salt							
Fluids (at least 8)							
Prenatal vitamin							

daily dozen diary

WEEK:	S	M	T	W	T	F	S
Protein foods (3)							
Calcium foods (4)							
Vitamin C foods (3)							
Green leafy/Yellows (3 to 4)							
Other fruits & vegetables (1 to 2)							
Whole grains & legumes (6 or more)							
Iron-rich foods (some daily)							
Fat (4)							
Salt							
Fluids (at least 8)							
Prenatal vitamin							

daily dozen diary

WEEK:	S	M	T	W	T	F	S
Protein foods (3)							
Calcium foods (4)							
Vitamin C foods (3)							
Green leafy/Yellows (3 to 4)							
Other fruits & vegetables (1 to 2)							
Whole grains & legumes (6 or more)							
Iron-rich foods (some daily)							
Fat (4)							
Salt							
Fluids (at least 8)							
Prenatal vitamin							

daily dozen diary

WEEK:	S	M	T	W	T	F	S
Protein foods (3)							
Calcium foods (4)							
Vitamin C foods (3)							
Green leafy/Yellows (3 to 4)							
Other fruits & vegetables (1 to 2)							
Whole grains & legumes (6 or more)							
Iron-rich foods (some daily)							
Fat (4)							
Salt							
Fluids (at least 8)							
Prenatal vitamin							

daily dozen diary

WEEK:	S	M	T	W	T	F	S
Protein foods (3)							
Calcium foods (4)							
Vitamin C foods (3)							
Green leafy/Yellows (3 to 4)							
Other fruits & vegetables (1 to 2)							
Whole grains & legumes (6 or more)							
Iron-rich foods (some daily)							
Fat (4)							
Salt							
Fluids (at least 8)							
Prenatal vitamin							

weight gain tracker

finding those pregnancy pounds piling on easily? Or are you struggling (thanks to morning sickness or aversions) to get that gain going? Whether your pregnancy weight gain has been in the fast lane, the slow lane, or somewhere in between, the best way to keep it on track is to keep track of it on this graph. Weigh yourself every week or two if you have a scale at home, then locate the number of weeks of pregnancy at the bottom of the graph and find your weight gain in pounds along the left side of the graph. Make a dot where the pounds meet the weeks. Play connect the dots to see your rate of change.

	FIRST TRIMESTER	SECOND TRIMESTER	THIRD TRIMESTER

WEIGHT GAIN (LBS.)

50
48
46
44
42
40
38
36
34
32
30
28
26
24
22
20
18
16
14
12
10
8
6
4
2
0

0 2 4 6 8 10 12 14   16 18 20 22 24 26 28   30 32 34 36 38 40 42

WEEKS

baby movement tracker

early in pregnancy, movements can be erratic (one day baby's kicking up a storm, next day all's quiet on the uterine front)—and that's fine. But from the 28th week on, you should hear (or rather feel) from your baby regularly—and that's a sign that all is well within. To make sure you do, check for fetal movement twice daily, morning and evening. You should be able to detect ten movements within a two-hour period, though most often you will get to ten in a much shorter time. Any kind of movement counts (not just kicks). Keep track below (you can make a check mark for each daily test, or record the time it took to reach 10 movements).

before you forget

Remember to record your reaction and that of your partner to feeling your baby move in the Journal section of this book.

WEEK 28	S	M	T	W	T	F	S
Morning							
Evening							

WEEK 29	S	M	T	W	T	F	S
Morning							
Evening							

WEEK 30	S	M	T	W	T	F	S
Morning							
Evening							

WEEK 31	S	M	T	W	T	F	S
Morning							
Evening							

WEEK 32	S	M	T	W	T	F	S
Morning							
Evening							

WEEK 33	S	M	T	W	T	F	S
Morning							
Evening							

WEEK 34	S	M	T	W	T	F	S
Morning							
Evening							

WEEK 35	S	M	T	W	T	F	S
Morning							
Evening							

WEEK 36	S	M	T	W	T	F	S
Morning							
Evening							

WEEK 37	S	M	T	W	T	F	S
Morning							
Evening							

WEEK 38	S	M	T	W	T	F	S
Morning							
Evening							

WEEK 39	S	M	T	W	T	F	S
Morning							
Evening							

WEEK 40	S	M	T	W	T	F	S
Morning							
Evening							

WEEK 41	S	M	T	W	T	F	S
Morning							
Evening							

WEEK 42	S	M	T	W	T	F	S
Morning							
Evening							

getting ready for labor and delivery

U se this section to take childbirth-class notes, to develop a birth plan to discuss with your practitioner, to figure out what to look for when you visit the hospital or birthing center, to itemize what you'll need to pack for the hospital or birthing center, and to list people to call when you go into labor or after you deliver.

childbirth education classes

t o make sure you retain what you learn in childbirth education class (and can apply it later on, when it counts), take notes.

Class name _____ Date _____

Instructor _____

Class notes _____

_____

_____

_____

Instructions _____

_____

_____

Homework _____

_____

Class name   Date

Instructor

Class notes

Instructions

Homework

Class name   Date

Instructor

Class notes

Instructions

Homework

Class name _____ Date _____

Instructor _____

Class notes _____

_____

_____

_____

Instructions _____

_____

Homework _____

Class name _____ Date _____

Instructor _____

Class notes _____

_____

_____

_____

Instructions _____

_____

Homework _____

_____

Class name _____ Date _____

Instructor _____

Class notes _____

_____

_____

_____

_____

_____

Instructions _____

_____

_____

Homework _____

Class name _____ Date _____

Instructor _____

Class notes _____

_____

_____

_____

_____

Instructions _____

_____

_____

Homework _____

_____

classmates we want to keep in touch with

NAME	PHONE	E-MAIL	DUE DATE

visiting the hospital or birthing center

even if you've been to a hospital before, you may not really know what to expect when it comes to the labor and delivery floor. Ditto a birthing center. To make sure you're clued in before that first contraction hits, schedule a visit to the hospital or birthing center where you plan to deliver. The more familiar you are with your surroundings, the more comfortable you'll be. Get ready to look and listen on your tour—and also to speak up. Go armed with a list of questions and jot down the answers before you forget them.

things to observe

Quickest driving route

Time it takes to arrive

Alternate route

Where to park

Overall impression of hospital or birthing center

Impressions of rooms

questions to ask

What standard procedures are done during labor?

Will I be able to labor, deliver, and recover in the same room?

What is the nurse-to-patient ratio?

Will someone be with me at all times?

What features are there in the birthing room (TV, music, dim lights, etc.)?

What is your policy on:

　Electronic fetal monitoring

　IVs

　Eating during labor

Do you have a squat bar?　　　　　　A birthing chair?

Do you have a labor tub?　　　　　　A shower?

Do you allow water births?

What is the hospital's C-section rate?

What is the hospital's VBAC rate?

What is the hospital's epidural rate?

Can my spouse and/or doula be with me at all times?

Even if I have a C-section?

How many people can I have with me during labor and delivery?

Can my spouse video the birth?

Are cell phones allowed?

Can I breastfeed right after my baby is born?

Is a pediatrician available immediately in case my baby needs one?

What routine tests will my baby get?

What routine vaccinations will my baby get?

What routine procedures will my baby undergo?

Do you have a NICU?

Is there a place for my partner to lie down during labor?

Can my partner stay with me in my postpartum room?

Will there be a place for him to sleep?

What are my rooming-in options with my baby?

Is a lactation consultant available?

What is your visitor policy?

What about for siblings?

How long can I stay after a vaginal birth?

How quickly can I be discharged?

How long can I stay after a C-section?

How quickly can I be discharged?

What is the average cost of a vaginal birth?

What is the average cost of a C-section?

Other questions

NOTES

my birth plan

Y ou know that your practitioner (and the staff at the hospital or birthing center) will have some say in what happens during your labor and delivery. But chances are, you'd also like some input into your birth experience. Luckily, you can have it—by setting up a birth plan. Use the pages below to explore your options, keeping in mind that since not all labors and deliveries go as planned, you might not be able to call all the shots in advance. Fill in as much—or as little—as you'd like on these pages. If you'd like, you can copy these pages and hand them out to your practitioner and the nurses on staff when you arrive for delivery.

birth philosophy

This birth plan expresses our desires and preferences for the birth of our baby. We have educated ourselves before making these choices, and we understand that there may be situations in which our choices may not be possible. In such instances:

☐ THE PRACTITIONER MAY MAKE THE NECESSARY DECISIONS FOR THE HEALTH AND SAFETY OF MOTHER AND BABY.

☐ WE ASK THAT THE PRACTITIONER DISCUSS WITH US ANY PROCEDURES OR MEDICATIONS PRIOR TO ADMINISTRATION AND THAT WE BE ALLOWED THE CHANCE TO QUESTION SUCH PROCEDURES BEFORE GIVING INFORMED CONSENT.

special situations

Please note that I:

☐ AM TRYING FOR A VBAC

☐ HAVE GESTATIONAL DIABETES

☐ HAVE PREECLAMPSIA

☐ HAVE RH INCOMPATIBILITY WITH THE BABY

☐ HAVE TESTED POSITIVE FOR GROUP B STREP

☐ OTHER

the environment (check all that apply)

I'd like these people to be in the room with me:

- ☐ MY PARTNER
- ☐ OUR PARENT(S)
- ☐ MY OTHER CHILDREN
- ☐ MY DOULA
- ☐ OTHER

Special things I'd like during labor:

- ☐ DIM LIGHTS
- ☐ MINIMAL INTERRUPTIONS
- ☐ MUSIC
- ☐ NO LOUD NOISES
- ☐ NO STUDENTS OR RESIDENTS CHECKING ON ME
- ☐ TO VIDEO AND TAKE PICTURES

- ☐
- ☐
- ☐
- ☐
- ☐
- ☐

the labor experience (check all that apply)

I hope to have a:

- ☐ VAGINAL DELIVERY
- ☐ CESAREAN SECTION

- ☐ VBAC
- ☐ WATER BIRTH

I'd like to wear my:

- ☐ CONTACTS
- ☐ GLASSES

I prefer:

- ☐ THAT MY PARTNER NOT BE SEPARATED FROM ME AT ANY STAGE OF CHILDBIRTH
- ☐ INFREQUENT VAGINAL EXAMS
- ☐ TO BE ABLE TO EAT DURING LABOR

☐ TO BE ABLE TO DRINK DURING LABOR

☐ TO STAY HYDRATED VIA CLEAR LIQUIDS AND ICE CHIPS

☐ NOT TO HAVE MY LABOR AUGMENTED AS LONG AS MY BABY AND I ARE FINE

☐ THAT MY MEMBRANES NOT BE ARTIFICIALLY RUPTURED

If my labor needs to be induced or augmented, I prefer:

☐ NATURAL METHODS (NIPPLE STIMULATION, FOR EXAMPLE)

☐ STRIPPING OF MEMBRANES

☐ PROSTAGLANDIN GEL

☐ PITOCIN

☐ BREAKING OF MEMBRANES

☐ OTHER

I'd like to spend the first stage of labor:

☐ IN A BATHTUB

☐ IN A SHOWER

☐ LYING DOWN

☐ SITTING UP

☐ WALKING AROUND

☐ OTHER

I do not want the following:

☐ ENEMA

☐ SHAVED PUBIC AREA

☐ IV LINE

☐ IV LINE, BUT A HEPARIN LOCK IS OK

☐ URINARY CATHETER

☐ OTHER

I'd like my baby to be monitored:

- ☐ CONTINUOUSLY
- ☐ INTERMITTENTLY
- ☐ INTERNALLY
- ☐ EXTERNALLY
- ☐ WITH A DOPPLER ONLY
- ☐ AT PRACTITIONER'S DISCRETION

I'd like to be given pain medication:

- ☐ ONLY IF I REQUEST IT. PLEASE DON'T OFFER IT TO ME.
- ☐ IF I SEEM UNCOMFORTABLE
- ☐ AS SOON AS POSSIBLE

I want to manage my pain in the following ways:

- ☐ BREATHING TECHNIQUES
- ☐ MEDITATION
- ☐ ACUPRESSURE
- ☐ ACUPUNCTURE
- ☐ DISTRACTION
- ☐ HYPNOSIS
- ☐ HYDROTHERAPY
- ☐ MASSAGE
- ☐ REFLEXOLOGY
- ☐ TENS
- ☐ EPIDURAL
- ☐ WALKING EPIDURAL
- ☐ DEMEROL
- ☐ I WANT TO DECIDE DURING LABOR
- ☐ OTHER

the delivery (check all that apply)

When pushing, I'd like to be in the following position:

- ☐ SQUATTING
- ☐ SEMIRECLINING
- ☐ SIDE-LYING
- ☐ LEANING ON MY SUPPORT PERSON
- ☐ USING PEOPLE FOR LEG SUPPORT
- ☐ USING FOOT PEDALS FOR LEG SUPPORT

☐ USING A BIRTHING BAR OVER ☐ IN A BATHTUB

THE BED FOR SUPPORT ☐ ON A BIRTHING STOOL

☐ ON HANDS AND KNEES ☐ LET ME DECIDE THEN

☐ STANDING ☐ OTHER

I'd also like to:

☐ PUSH WHEN I FEEL LIKE IT (SPONTANEOUS PUSHING)

☐ PUSH WHEN DIRECTED BY NURSES OR MY COACH

☐ HAVE NO TIME LIMITS ON PUSHING (AS LONG AS MY BABY AND I ARE FINE)

☐ HAVE THE EPIDURAL WEAR OFF BEFORE PUSHING

☐ CONTINUE WITH A FULL-DOSE EPIDURAL WHILE PUSHING

☐ SEE THE BIRTH IN A MIRROR

☐ TOUCH MY BABY'S HEAD AS IT CROWNS

☐ OTHER

About an episiotomy:

☐ USE PERINEAL MASSAGE, WARM COMPRESSES, AND POSITIONING FIRST

☐ I'D RATHER RISK A TEAR THAN HAVE AN EPISIOTOMY

☐ I'D RATHER HAVE AN EPISIOTOMY THAN RISK A TEAR

☐ HAVE AN EPISIOTOMY ONLY AS A LAST RESORT

☐ HAVE AN EPISIOTOMY AT THE PRACTITIONER'S DISCRETION

☐ USE NO LOCAL ANESTHESIA; I PREFER A PRESSURE EPISIOTOMY

☐ USE LOCAL ANESTHESIA ONLY DURING REPAIR

If an assisted birth becomes necessary, I'd rather:

☐ HAVE FORCEPS

☐ HAVE VACUUM EXTRACTION

☐ HAVE IT BE AT THE PRACTITIONER'S DISCRETION

Delivering the baby:

☐ MY PARTNER WOULD LIKE TO CATCH THE BABY

☐ I WOULD LIKE TO HELP CATCH THE BABY

☐ MY PARTNER WOULD LIKE TO SUCTION THE BABY

If a cesarean becomes necessary:

☐ I WOULD LIKE TO BE CONSCIOUS

☐ I WOULD LIKE MY PARTNER TO BE WITH ME AT ALL TIMES

☐ I WOULD LIKE THE SCREEN LOWERED SO I CAN SEE THE BABY COMING OUT

☐ I WOULD LIKE TO BE ABLE TO TOUCH THE BABY; PLEASE LEAVE MY HANDS FREE

☐ PLEASE EXPLAIN THE SURGERY TO ME AS IT HAPPENS

☐ OTHER

after delivery (check all that apply)

The umbilical cord:

☐ MY PARTNER WOULD LIKE TO CUT THE UMBILICAL CORD

☐ WAIT UNTIL THE UMBILICAL CORD STOPS PULSATING BEFORE CUTTING

☐ I HAVE MADE ARRANGEMENTS FOR DONATION OF THE CORD BLOOD

☐ I HAVE MADE ARRANGEMENTS TO PRIVATELY BANK THE CORD BLOOD

The placenta:

☐ I WOULD LIKE TO DELIVER THE PLACENTA SPONTANEOUSLY AND UNASSISTED

☐ I WOULD LIKE TO SEE THE PLACENTA AFTER IT IS DELIVERED

☐ I DO NOT WANT PITOCIN TO BE ADMINISTERED AFTER DELIVERY

I would like to hold my baby:

- ☐ IMMEDIATELY AFTER DELIVERY; PLEASE PLACE THE BABY ON MY ABDOMEN
- ☐ AFTER SUCTIONING
- ☐ AFTER WEIGHING
- ☐ AFTER HE OR SHE IS WIPED CLEAN AND SWADDLED
- ☐ BEFORE EYEDROPS OR OINTMENT ARE ADMINISTERED
- ☐ OTHER

I would like to breastfeed:

- ☐ IMMEDIATELY AFTER DELIVERY
- ☐ BEFORE EYEDROPS OR OINTMENT ARE ADMINISTERED
- ☐ LATER
- ☐ NOT AT ALL

I would like family members to:

- ☐ BE ABLE TO JOIN US AND THE BABY IN THE ROOM RIGHT AFTER DELIVERY
- ☐ BE ABLE TO JOIN US AND THE BABY IN THE ROOM LATER
- ☐ SEE THE BABY IN THE NURSERY ONLY

Newborn procedures:

- ☐ I'D LIKE MY BABY'S MEDICAL EXAM TO BE PERFORMED IN MY PRESENCE
- ☐ I'D LIKE MY BABY'S MEDICAL EXAM TO BE PERFORMED ONLY AFTER WE'VE HAD A CHANCE TO BOND
- ☐ I DON'T NEED TO BE THERE
- ☐ MY PARTNER WOULD LIKE TO BE THERE
- ☐ I'D LIKE MY BABY TO HAVE A HEEL STICK FOR NEWBORN SCREENING TESTS
- ☐ I DO NOT WANT MY BABY TO RECEIVE A VITAMIN K SHOT
- ☐ I'D LIKE TO HAVE MY BABY TESTED FOR METABOLIC DISORDERS. I HAVE ARRANGED FOR SUCH TESTING.

first hours (check all that apply)

My baby's first bath:

- ☐ I'D LIKE TO BE THERE
- ☐ I DON'T NEED TO BE THERE
- ☐ MY PARTNER WOULD LIKE TO BE PRESENT
- ☐ I PREFER TO GIVE THE FIRST BATH

Feeding:

- ☐ I PLAN TO EXCLUSIVELY BREASTFEED
- ☐ I PLAN TO FORMULA FEED
- ☐ I PLAN TO BREASTFEED AND FORMULA FEED
- ☐ I PLAN TO FEED ON DEMAND
- ☐ I PLAN TO FEED ON A SCHEDULE
- ☐ I WOULD LIKE THE HELP OF A LACTATION SPECIALIST

Please do not offer my baby any of the following:

- ☐ FORMULA
- ☐ SUGAR WATER
- ☐ PACIFIER

I'd like my baby to be:

- ☐ IN MY ROOM 24 HOURS
- ☐ IN MY ROOM ONLY DURING THE DAY
- ☐ IN MY ROOM ONLY WHEN I'M AWAKE
- ☐ IN THE NURSERY EXCEPT AT FEEDING TIME
- ☐ OTHER

I'd like my partner to:

- ☐ HAVE UNLIMITED VISITATION
- ☐ HAVE LIMITED VISITATION
- ☐ SLEEP IN MY ROOM

I'd like family members to:

☐ VISIT ONLY AT THESE TIMES   ☐ HAVE UNLIMITED VISITATION

I'd like baby's older siblings to:

☐ VISIT ONLY AT THESE TIMES   ☐ HAVE UNLIMITED VISITATION

If my baby's a boy:

☐ I WANT HIM CIRCUMCISED

☐ I WANT HIM CIRCUMCISED WITH ANESTHESIA

☐ I DON'T WANT HIM CIRCUMCISED

☐ I'D LIKE TO BE PRESENT FOR THE CIRCUMCISION

☐ MY PARTNER WOULD LIKE TO BE PRESENT

I'd like my stay in the hospital/birthing center to be:

☐ AS SHORT AS POSSIBLE

☐ AS LONG AS POSSIBLE

☐ I'D LIKE TO DECIDE AFTER THE BIRTH

I'd like the following medications to be offered to me after delivery as needed:

☐ EXTRA-STRENGTH ACETAMINOPHEN   ☐ STOOL SOFTENER

☐ PERCOSET   ☐ LAXATIVE

If my baby needs special care, I'd like to:

☐ ACCOMPANY OR HAVE MY PARTNER ACCOMPANY THE BABY TO THE NICU

   OR ANOTHER FACILITY

☐ BREASTFEED OR PROVIDE EXPRESSED BREASTMILK FOR MY BABY

☐ HOLD MY BABY WHENEVER POSSIBLE

☐ OTHER

choosing a birth doula

a doula (from the ancient Greek word meaning "woman servant") can provide you with the extra support (and hand-holding and brow wiping) that can make all the difference—not only during birth but also before and after. Her experience will also come in handy. In gauging that experience, as well as her other qualifications, you'll want to interview wisely. (Make copies of these pages if you're planning to interview more than one doula.) For a postpartum doula interview, see page 268.

doula interview

Name

Address

Phone

Recommended by

Agency, if any

What are your fees and what payment options do you offer?

Why did you become a doula?

Where did you learn to be a doula?

Do you have any official certifications?

What do you like best about your job?

How long have you been doing this?

How many clients do you have?

About how many births have you attended?

What are your birthing philosophies (for example, your opinion on epidurals)?

What services do you typically provide?

Will you be on call at all times?

How do I contact you before I go into labor?

How do I contact you when labor begins?

If you're unavailable, who fills in for you?

When I go into labor, do you meet me at home or at the place of birth?

Do you attend home births?

Do you have another client due around my due date?

Have you ever worked with my obstetrician/midwife?

What was that experience like?

What support services will you provide if I need a C-section?

Do you provide any postpartum services? (For more questions to ask a postpartum doula, see page 268.)

Can you provide me with references?

packing my bag

u nless you're giving birth at home, you'll want to have a bag packed and ready to go several weeks before your due date (yes, weeks—just in case your baby decides to make an early appearance). Pack more than you think you'll need (you'll end up needing whatever you don't end up packing), but also remember to tailor this list to your needs.

labor gear

☐ THIS BOOK, AND PENS OR PENCILS TO FILL IN THE BLANKS

☐ YOUR BIRTH PLAN (several copies, so all staff on all shifts can get one)

☐ STOPWATCH OR CELL PHONE TIMER TO TIME CONTRACTIONS

☐ MASSAGE OILS OR LOTIONS

☐ YOUR FAVORITE PILLOW

☐ A CLIP OR SCRUNCHIE TO KEEP YOUR HAIR OUT OF YOUR FACE (if you have long hair)

☐ SUGARLESS CANDIES OR LOLLIPOPS TO KEEP YOUR MOUTH MOIST

☐ BACKRUB TOOLS: A TENNIS BALL, PLASTIC ROLLING PIN, OR AN ACTUAL MASSAGER

☐ SNACKS FOR LABOR (your own snacks will be limited and must be approved by your practitioner; your partner should pack sandwiches and other sustaining nibbles so he doesn't have to leave your side to find something to eat)

☐ DIVERSIONS FOR A LONG LABOR: iPOD, E-READER, SMARTPHONE, PUZZLES, MAGAZINES, BOOKS, A DECK OF CARDS, LAPTOP

☐ ANY MEMENTOS YOU'LL WANT, SUCH AS FAMILY PHOTOS

☐ A *WHO TO CALL* LIST (see pages 241–242) AND A PREPAID PHONE CARD OR CALLING CARD (in case the hospital doesn't allow cell phones)

☐ CAMERA AND/OR CELL PHONE WITH CAMERA—even if you don't want to capture your labor and delivery experience, you'll definitely want to capture your baby's image, and someone in the room will be happy to take your first family portrait

personal items

- [ ] A BABY BOOK FOR RECORDING EVERYTHING
- [ ] TOOTHBRUSH, TOOTHPASTE, AND MOUTHWASH [ ] HAIRBRUSH AND COMB
- [ ] SHOWER GEL, FACE WASH, SHAMPOO, CONDITIONER, MAKEUP, MOISTURIZER (and whatever else it takes to make you feel human again after delivery)
- [ ] EXTRA-ABSORBENT MAXI-PADS (the hospital will provide some, but you might want to use the brand you're most comfortable with)
- [ ] NONPERISHABLE SNACKS FOR AFTER DELIVERY (such as dried fruit and nuts and granola bars; don't count on the hospital or birthing center to provide them in the middle of the night)
- [ ] CHAMPAGNE OR SPARKLING CIDER (you'll want to celebrate)
- [ ] A BABY-CARE BOOK, LIKE *WHAT TO EXPECT THE FIRST YEAR* (if you want to lug it and think you'll have a chance to look at it)

clothes

- [ ] EXTRA PAIRS OF UNDERWEAR SUITABLE FOR WEARING WITH MAXI-PADS (no thongs, please) AND A NURSING BRA
- [ ] NIGHTGOWN OR PJS, SOCKS, AND SLIPPERS
- [ ] COMFORTABLE OUTFIT TO HEAD HOME IN (remember, you'll still look six months pregnant, so plan accordingly)
- [ ] GOING-HOME OUTFIT FOR BABY (don't forget socks or booties and a receiving blanket, plus extra layers if it's cold)
- [ ] A FEW DIAPERS (although the hospital will probably provide them)

other essentials

- [ ] REAR-FACING INFANT CAR SEAT (This won't go in the suitcase with you, of course, but when it comes time to take your newborn home, your partner should know how to find it quickly and install it correctly. Better still, install it in advance so you're ready to roll after you're both checked out.)

who to call
when labor begins

Keep these telephone numbers handy (and stored in your cell phone) so when that first contraction strikes, you won't need to frantically flip through your address book (or try to remember your partner's cell phone number while trying to remember which breathing techniques to use).

PARTNER OR LABOR COACH: HOME

WORK

CELL

	NAME	PHONE
Practitioner		
Doula		
Hospital or birthing center		
Your parents		
Partner's parents		
Your siblings		
Partner's siblings		
Babysitter (for other children)		
Neighbors/Friends/Coworkers		
Cab company		
Other		

who to call after delivery

	NAME	PHONE
Pediatrician		
Health insurance company		
Doula/Baby nurse		
Lactation specialist		
Clergy		
Diaper service		
Store deliveries (crib, layette, etc.)		

family members, friends, coworkers

NAME	PHONE	E-MAIL

getting ready for baby

it's a good thing babies take so long to grow—because getting ready for them takes so long, too. From the shopping to the decorating, from the financial planning (so you can afford all that shopping and decorating) to the festivities to celebrate baby's arrival, preparing your nest for your little fledgling will take plenty of time—and plenty of effort. Most of all, it will take plenty of organization as you try to keep track of everything you need to buy and get done before D-day. This section is for keeping track so you can get it all done—and done in time.

choosing baby's name

a word to the wise parent: Don't leave this important decision for the last minute. Though you might want to hold off on finalizing until you've held your little bundle in your arms (sometimes babies name themselves), you should try to at least have your name pool narrowed down by D-day. Sometimes writing the candidates on paper, along with their meanings and the reasons for considering them, makes it easier to evaluate and compare them. Use these pages for that purpose in the months before delivery.

girls' names

FIRST	MIDDLE	MEANING	WHY WE LIKE IT

girls' names (continued)

FIRST	MIDDLE	MEANING	WHY WE LIKE IT

boys' names

FIRST	MIDDLE	MEANING	WHY WE LIKE IT

baby gear

U se these pages to keep an organized (and ever updated) list of what you have, what you want, and what you'll need—now and eventually—when it comes to baby gear. For information on choosing baby gear, see *What to Expect the First Year.*

baby's wardrobe

ITEM	HAVE	NEED	SOURCE
3–10 undershirts/onesies			
4–7 stretchies with feet			
1–2 two-piece outfits			
3–6 rompers			
3–6 nightgowns with elastic bottoms			
2–3 blanket sleepers			
1–3 sweaters			
1–3 hats			
1 bunting or snowsuit			
2–3 pairs booties/socks			
3 washable bibs			
3–4 waterproof pants, diaper covers, or diaper wraps, if using cloth diapers			

baby's linens

ITEM	HAVE	NEED	SOURCE
3–4 fitted sheets for bassinet, crib, and/or carriage			
2–6 waterproof pads			
2 mattress pads			
2 blankets for stroller or car seat *(Note: avoid using while baby is sleeping because of the risk of SIDS)*			
2–3 terrycloth towels			
2–3 terry washcloths			
12 cloth diapers (burping cloths)			
2–5 receiving blankets			
1–2 packages disposable diapers (newborn size)			
2–5 dozen cloth diapers, or all-in-ones (if you'll be using)			

baby's grooming needs

ITEM	HAVE	NEED	SOURCE
Baby soap/bath liquid			
No-tears baby shampoo			
Baby oil			
Baby powder, optional			
Diaper rash ointment/cream			
Petroleum jelly			
Cleansing wipes			
Cotton balls			
Baby nail scissors or clippers			
Baby brush and comb			
Diaper pins (if using cloth diapers)			

baby's medicine cabinet

ITEM	HAVE	NEED	SOURCE
Liquid infant acetaminophen (Tylenol)			
Antibiotic ointment or cream			
Hydrogen peroxide			
Calamine lotion			
Hydrocortisone cream (0.5%)			
Rehydration fluid			
Sunscreen			
Rubbing alcohol			
Calibrated spoon, dropper, and/or oral syringe			
Sterile bandages			
Tweezers			
Nasal aspirator			
Digital thermometer			
Tongue depressors			

baby's feeding supplies

ITEM	HAVE	NEED	SOURCE
4 four-ounce bottles and 10–12 eight-ounce bottles, if bottle feeding			
Utensils for formula preparation, if bottle feeding			
Formula			
4–6 eight-ounce bottles, if breastfeeding			
Breast pump, if breastfeeding			
Bags to store breastmilk			
Pacifier, if using			

baby's outing gear

ITEM	HAVE	NEED	SOURCE
Stroller and/or carriage			
Infant safety seat			
Baby carrier or sling			
Diaper bag			

baby's nursery gear

ITEM	HAVE	NEED	SOURCE
Bassinet or cradle			
Crib			
Crib mattress			
Changing space			
Diaper pail			
Baby tub			
Infant seat			
Rocking chair or glider			
Baby monitor			
Baby swing			
Night-light			
Portable crib			

for when baby's older

ITEM	HAVE	NEED	SOURCE
High chair			
Portable feeding seat			
Play yard			
Safety gate			
Stationary entertainer			

other

ITEM	HAVE	NEED	SOURCE

comparison shopping

Item

Store/Salesperson   Phone

Make/Style

Size   Color   Price

Delivery/Availability

Features

Item

Store/Salesperson   Phone

Make/Style

Size   Color   Price

Delivery/Availability

Features

Item

Store/Salesperson   Phone

Make/Style

Size   Color   Price

Delivery/Availability

Features

Item

Store/Salesperson   Phone

Make/Style

Size   Color   Price

Delivery/Availability

Features

Item

Store/Salesperson   Phone

Make/Style

Size   Color   Price

Delivery/Availability

Features

Item

Store/Salesperson   Phone

Make/Style

Size   Color   Price

Delivery/Availability

Features

Item

Store/Salesperson   Phone

Make/Style

Size   Color   Price

Delivery/Availability

Features

Item

Store/Salesperson   Phone

Make/Style

Size   Color   Price

Delivery/Availability

Features

Item

Store/Salesperson   Phone

Make/Style

Size   Color   Price

Delivery/Availability

Features

decorating the nursery

Will it be pink bunnies or blue choo-choos? A three-ring circus or a stellar solar system? Girlish gingham or boyish plaids? With so many cute options (and, possibly, so little time before the paint has to be dry), you may be a little overwhelmed by the prospect of decorating the room your baby will soon be calling home. However you decide to tackle the project, it'll help to keep notes. Use these pages to tie it all together.

option #1

Nursery theme

Paint colors

Wallpaper

Murals or decals

Fabric

Accessories

PLACE FABRIC

SWATCHES AND

PAINT CHIPS

HERE

option #2

Nursery theme

Paint colors

Wallpaper

Murals or decals

Fabric

Accessories

PLACE FABRIC SWATCHES AND

PAINT CHIPS HERE

option #3

Nursery theme

Paint colors

Wallpaper

Murals or decals

Fabric

Accessories

PLACE FABRIC SWATCHES AND

PAINT CHIPS HERE

baby registry

b aby registries are available at most stores that sell baby products, as well as online. Registering will ensure that you get what you want—and the right amount of what you want—so you can spend the early postpartum days enjoying your baby instead of exchanging and returning baby gifts.

Store _____ Registry ID number _____

Web site _____ Username/password _____

Store phone _____ Contact person _____

Items on registry _____

_____

_____

_____

NOTES _____

_____

Store _____ Registry ID number _____

Web site _____ Username/password _____

Store phone _____ Contact person _____

Items on registry _____

_____

_____

_____

NOTES _____

_____

Store   Registry ID number

Web site   Username/password

Store phone   Contact person

Items on registry

NOTES

Store   Registry ID number

Web site   Username/password

Store phone   Contact person

Items on registry

NOTES

my baby shower

Your baby shower (or showers, if you're lucky enough to get more than one) is bound to be memorable—but just to be on the safe side, fill in these blanks as soon as you get home.

Date

Place

Hosted by

Theme/decorations

Food served

Games played

Entertainment

Gift bags given

Memorable moments

Funniest moment

Most sentimental moment

GUEST	GIFT	THANK-YOU

my baby shower

Date

Place

Hosted by

Theme/decorations

Food served

Games played

Entertainment

Gift bags given

Memorable moments

Funniest moment

Most sentimental moment

GUEST	GIFT	THANK-YOU

birth announcement list

Sure, you won't be alerting the media (and a thousand of your closest friends and family) about your baby's arrival until it actually happens. But you might want to save yourself some time (a precious postpartum commodity, as you'll find) by getting your birth-announcement list together now.

NAME	ADDRESS	E-MAIL

NAME	ADDRESS	E-MAIL

NAME	ADDRESS	E-MAIL

NAME	ADDRESS	E-MAIL

NAME	ADDRESS	E-MAIL

choosing a pediatrician

Since your child's pediatrician will be a very important person in your life over the coming years, you'll want someone you like, someone you can trust (and feel comfortable calling at 2 A.M.), and someone who sees eye-to-eye with you when it comes to parenting philosophies (though keep in mind that yours will evolve). To make sure you're on the same page as the pediatricians you're considering, schedule a consulation and ask these or other questions you may have. (You can make copies of these pages if you're planning to interview more than one pediatrician.) Some of the office protocol and business questions are best answered by office personnel.

pediatrician interview

Name

Address

Phone   Fax

E-mail address

Office hours   Typical waiting time

Call hours

What are your fees?

What payment options do you offer?

Do you accept my health insurance?

How long have you been in practice?

Where did you receive your training?

Affiliated hospital/birthing center

Address and phone

Who will answer my questions when I call?

Can you answer questions by e-mail?

Type of practice (solo, group, HMO, etc.)

If group, will my baby always be seen by the same doctor?

Will I have a choice of doctor?

Is a nurse practitioner part of practice?

When would my child see the nurse practitioner?

Who fills in when the doctor isn't available?

What protocol is followed in emergencies?

What protocol is followed with sick children (e.g., separate office hours or

waiting room)?

Your attitude to issues I care about:

  breastfeeding

  circumcision

  nutrition

  vegetarianism

  antibiotic use

  vaccinations

  other

My observations:

choosing a baby nurse or postpartum doula

looking for another pair of hands to help free yours up in the weeks after baby's born? Consider hiring a baby nurse or postpartum doula (who's different from a birth doula) to pick up the slack (and, hopefully, the house). But don't do the hiring without doing your homework. Interview a few candidates first to find the right match. Keep in mind that baby nurses usually confine their help to baby care, while a doula is more apt to help *you*— with cleaning, shopping, cooking, and so on. (You can make copies of these pages if you're planning to interview more than one child-care helper.)

baby nurse or postpartum doula interview

Name

Address

Phone   E-mail

Recommended by

Agency, if any

Are you available at the time of my due date?

What are your fees?

What days and hours are you available?

Are you available evenings and/or weekends?

Do you sleep in or out?

What training and experience do you have?

Are you certified in infant CPR?

What is your health and TB status?

What do you like best about your job?

How do you feel about:

☐ breastfeeding

☐ on-demand feeding

☐ scheduled feedings

☐ nap and sleep schedules

☐ other

Do you have a driver's license?

Are you comfortable with pets (if applicable)?

Are you willing to do:

☐ cooking

☐ heavy cleaning

☐ light cleaning

☐ laundry

☐ care for older siblings

Can you provide me with references?

NOTES

after the baby is born

t hought you had a lot to keep track of when you were expecting? That was nothing, Mom! Now that baby has arrived, life will be more joyful than ever—but also, more complicated. Use this section to start keeping track of those postpartum details—from the doctor's instructions you're afraid you'll forget to those baby celebrations you'll always want to remember. Those—and the truckloads of baby gifts ("Now, who did that romper with the blue teddy bears on it come from again?").

postpartum care instructions

y ou're probably more than preoccupied with how to care for your newborn, especially if you're a newbie parent. But don't forget that you'll need some care, too, in the postpartum period. Write down your practitioner's (and the nurses') instructions here so you won't forget a thing.

Perineal care

Incision care (if applicable)

Pain relief

Stool softener

Medication

Breast care

Breastfeeding

Diet

Other

baby care instructions

O f course, you're hanging on the doctor's and nurses' every word as they explain the basics of caring for your newborn. But will you remember a word they said once you're home and have no call light by your bed? You will if you write the instructions down here.

Feeding

Bathing

Cord care

Diaper care

Care of circumcision, if applicable

Other instructions

When to call for first well-baby visit

NOTES

baby gifts

When the packages start rolling in, it'll be hard to remember which came from whom. Keep track of the incoming here.

FROM	GIFT	THANK-YOU

FROM	GIFT	THANK-YOU

special celebrations

Whether it's a baptism or a bris or a welcome baby party you've got planned, if you've decided to celebrate the arrival of your little one with a big bash, you'll want to record all the details.

Event

Date

Baby's age

Menu

Decorations/Theme

Guest list

How I felt

What my baby wore

What I wore

How my baby reacted

Memorable moments

PLACE PHOTO HERE

before my six-week checkup

With lots of peculiar changes going on in your body, you'll likely find a reason to call your practitioner during those first six postpartum weeks. Keep a record here.

calls made to practitioner

Date called

Reason

Practitioner's response/instructions

Date called

Reason

Practitioner's response/instructions

Date called

Reason

Practitioner's response/instructions

questions to ask at the next visit

my six-week checkup

finally—your opportunity to ask all those questions you didn't have time to call about during the last six weeks! Plus, a chance to find out how much weight you've lost since you were pregnant. . . .

Appointment date _____ Time _____

Practitioner _____

Weight _____

Blood pressure _____

Other tests _____

_____

Pap smear _____

Method of birth control selected, if any _____

Prescriptions, if any _____

_____

_____

Practitioner's instructions on: _____

  Sex: _____

_____

  Weight loss/diet: _____

_____

  Exercise: _____

_____

  Breastfeeding: _____

_____

Other:

Next appointment

NOTES

P9-DNL-848

A Writer's Reference

SIXTH EDITION

A Writer's Reference

Diana Hacker

Contributing Authors

Nancy Sommers
Tom Jehn
Jane Rosenzweig
Harvard University

Contributing ESL Specialist

Marcy Carbajal Van Horn
Santa Fe Community College

BEDFORD / ST. MARTIN'S   Boston ◆ New York

For Bedford/St. Martin's

Executive Editor: Michelle M. Clark
Senior Production Editor: Anne Noonan
Senior Production Supervisor: Joe Ford
Senior Marketing Manager: John Swanson
Associate Editors: Amy Hurd Gershman and Mara Weible
Editorial Assistant: Jennifer Lyford
Assistant Production Editor: Amy Derjue
Copyeditor: Barbara G. Flanagan
Text Design: Claire Seng-Niemoeller
Cover Design: Donna Lee Dennison
Composition: Monotype, LLC
Printing and Binding: R.R. Donnelley & Sons Company

President: Joan E. Feinberg
Editorial Director: Denise B. Wydra
Editor in Chief: Karen S. Henry
Director of Marketing: Karen Melton Soeltz
Director of Editing, Design, and Production: Marcia Cohen
Managing Editor: Elizabeth M. Schaaf

Library of Congress Control Number: 2006926009

Copyright © 2007 by Bedford/St. Martin's

All rights reserved. No part of this book may be reproduced, stored in a retrieval system, or transmitted in any form or by any means, electronic, mechanical, photocopying, recording, or otherwise, except as may be expressly permitted by the applicable copyright statutes or in writing by the Publisher.

Manufactured in the United States of America.

1   0   9   8   7
f   e   d   c

For information, write: Bedford/St. Martin's, 75 Arlington Street, Boston, MA 02116 (617-399-4000)

ISBN-10: 0–312–45025–7
ISBN-13: 978–0–312–45025–0

ACKNOWLEDGMENTS

Scott Adams, "Dilbert and the Way of the Weasel." Copyright © 2000 by United Features Syndicate. Reprinted with permission of United Media.
American Heritage Dictionary, definition for "regard" from *The American Heritage Dictionary of the English Language, Fourth Edition.* Copyright © 2000 by Houghton Mifflin Company. Reprinted with permission.

Acknowledgments and copyrights are continued at the back of the book on page 509, which constitutes an extension of the copyright page. It is a violation of the law to reproduce these selections by any means whatsoever without the written permission of the copyright holder.

How to use this book

A Writer's Reference is designed to save you time. As you can see, the book lies flat, making it easy to consult while you are revising and editing a draft. And the book's twelve section dividers will lead you quickly to the information you need.

Here are brief descriptions of the book's major reference aids, followed by a chart summarizing the content of the book's companion Web site.

THE MENU SYSTEM.   The main menu inside the front cover displays the book's contents as briefly and simply as possible. Each of the twelve sections in the main menu leads you to a color-coded tabbed divider, on the back of which you will find a more detailed menu. Let's say you have a question about the proper use of commas between items in a series. Your first step is to scan the main menu, where you will find the comma listed as the first item in section P (Punctuation). Next flip the book open to the blue tabbed divider marked P. Now consult the detailed menu for the precise subsection (P1-c) and the exact page number.

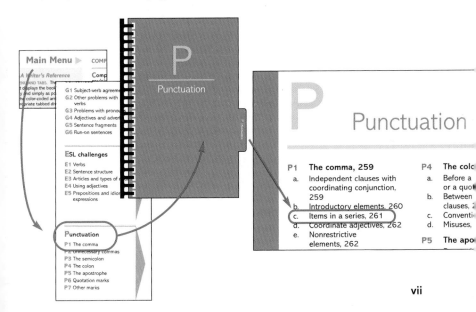

P   Punctuation

Punctuation

vii

DETAILED MENU (inside the back cover). A menu more detailed than the main menu appears inside the back cover.

CODES AND REVISION SYMBOLS. Some instructors mark student papers with the codes given on the main menu and detailed menus — section numbers such as S1 or G3-d. When you are revising an essay marked with codes, tracking down information is simple. When you see G3-d, for example, flip to the G tab — and then let the blue tabs at the tops of the pages lead you to G3-d, clear advice about when to use *who* and *whom*. If your instructor uses an abbreviation such as *dm* or *cs* instead of a number, consult the list of revision symbols on the next to last page of the book. There you will find the name of the problem (*dangling modifier*; *comma splice*) and the section number that will help you solve the problem.

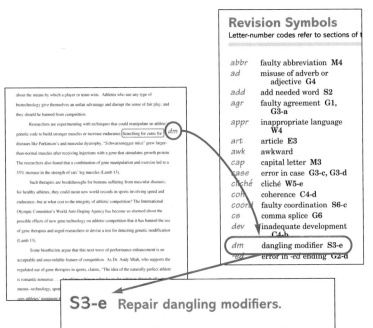

Revision Symbols

Letter-number codes refer to sections of

abbr	faulty abbreviation **M4**
ad	misuse of adverb or adjective **G4**
add	add needed word **S2**
agr	faulty agreement **G1, G3-a**
appr	inappropriate language **W4**
art	article **E3**
awk	awkward
cap	capital letter **M3**
case	error in case **G3-c, G3-d**
cliché	cliché **W5-e**
coh	coherence **C4-d**
coord	faulty coordination **S6-c**
cs	comma splice **G6**
dev	inadequate development **C4-b**
dm	dangling modifier **S3-e**
-ed	error in *-ed* ending **G2-d**

about the means by which a player or team wins. Athletes who use any type of biotechnology give themselves an unfair advantage and disrupt the sense of fair play, and they should be banned from competition.

Researchers are experimenting with techniques that could manipulate an athlete's genetic code to build stronger muscles or increase endurance. Searching for cures for diseases like Parkinson's and muscular dystrophy, "Schwarzenegger mice" grew larger-than-normal muscles after receiving injections with a gene that stimulates growth protein. The researchers also found that a combination of gene manipulation and exercise led to a 35% increase in the strength of rats' leg muscles (Lamb 13).

Such therapies are breakthroughs for humans suffering from muscular diseases; for healthy athletes, they could mean new world records in sports involving speed and endurance—but at what cost to the integrity of athletic competition? The International Olympic Committee's World Anti-Doping Agency has become so alarmed about the possible effects of new gene technology on athletic competition that it has banned the use of gene therapies and urged researchers to devise a test for detecting genetic modification (Lamb 13).

Some bioethicists argue that this next wave of performance enhancement is an acceptable and unavoidable feature of competition. As Dr. Andy Miah, who supports the regulated use of gene therapies in sports, claims, "The idea of the naturally perfect athlete is romantic nonsense. . . .

S3-e Repair dangling modifiers.

A dangling modifier fails to refer logically to any tence. Dangling modifiers are easy to repair, but t to recognize, especially in your own writing.

RULES, EXPLANATIONS, AND EXAMPLES. Once you use a code to find a section, such as G1-b, the text presents three main types of help to solve your writing problem. The section number is accompanied by a rule, which is often a revision strategy. The rule is followed by a clear, brief explanation and, in some sections, by one or more hand-edited examples.

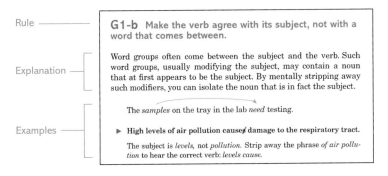

Rule

G1-b Make the verb agree with its subject, not with a word that comes between.

Explanation

Word groups often come between the subject and the verb. Such word groups, usually modifying the subject, may contain a noun that at first appears to be the subject. By mentally stripping away such modifiers, you can isolate the noun that is in fact the subject.

The *samples* on the tray in the lab *need* testing.

Examples

▶ High levels of air pollution cause damage to the respiratory tract.

The subject is *levels,* not *pollution.* Strip away the phrase *of air pollution* to hear the correct verb: *levels cause.*

THE INDEX. If you aren't sure what topic to choose from the main menu, consult the index at the back of the book. For example, you may not realize that the issue of whether to use *has* or *have* is a matter of subject-verb agreement (G1 on the main menu). In that case, simply look up "*has* vs. *have*" in the index. The boldface letter in the index entry leads you to the tabbed section G, and the page numbers pinpoint the specific page numbers in G. In addition, a cross-reference suggests another helpful index entry, "Subject-verb agreement."

Each index entry includes a reference to a tab letter and a page number.

THE GLOSSARY OF USAGE.   When in doubt about the correct use of a particular word (such as *affect* and *effect* or *among* and *between*), flip to section W1 and consult the alphabetically arranged glossary for the word in question. If the word you are looking for isn't in the glossary of usage, it may be in the index.

The glossary of
usage begins
on page 123.

Glossary of usage **W1**   127

censor, censure   *Censor* means "to remove or suppress material considered objectionable." *Censure* means "to criticize severely." *The school's policy of censoring books has been censured by the media.*

cite, site   *Cite* means "to quote as an authority or example." *Site* is usually a noun meaning "a particular place." *He cited the zoning law in his argument against the proposed site of the gas station.* Locations on the Internet are usually referred to as *sites*. *The library's Web site improves every week.*

climactic, climatic   *Climactic* is derived from *climax*, the point of greatest intensity in a series or progression of events. *Climatic* is derived from *climate* and refers to meteorological conditions. *The climactic period in the dinosaurs' reign was reached just before severe climatic conditions brought on an ice age.*

THE DIRECTORIES TO DOCUMENTATION MODELS.   When you are writing a research paper, you don't need to memorize technical details about handling citations or constructing a list of works you have cited. Instead, you can rely on one of the book's directories to documentation models to help you find examples of the types of citations you will need to provide in your paper. If you are using the Modern Language Association (MLA) system of documentation, flip the book open to the tabbed section marked MLA and then scan the tab menu to find the appropriate directory. If you are using the American Psychological Association (APA) or the *Chicago Manual of Style* (CMS) system, scan the menu on the tab marked APA/CMS.

The directory
to MLA works
cited models
begins on
page 379.

Directory to MLA works cited models

GENERAL GUIDELINES FOR LISTING AUTHORS

1. Single author, 380
2. Multiple authors, 380
3. Corporate author, 381
4. Unknown author, 381
5. Two or more works by the same author, 381

BOOKS

6. Basic format for a book, 382
7. Author with an editor, 382
8. Author with a translator, 382
9. Editor, 382
10. Work in an anthology, 382
11. Edition other than the first, 384
12. Multivolume work, 384
13. Encyclopedia or dictionary entry, 384
14. Sacred text, 385

31. Work from a service such as *InfoTrac*, 391
32. Article in an online periodical, 394
33. An entire Weblog (blog), 395
34. An entry in a Weblog (blog), 395
35. CD-ROM, 395
36. E-mail, 397
37. Posting to an online list, forum, or group, 397
38. Posting to a MUD or a MOO, 398

MULTIMEDIA SOURCES (INCLUDING ONLINE VERSIONS)

39. Work of art, 398
40. Cartoon, 398
41. Advertisement, 398
42. Map or chart, 398

COMPANION WEB SITE.   The following chart describes student resources available on the book's companion Web site.

ON THE WEB > dianahacker.com/writersref

▶ Writing exercises

Interactive exercises on topics such as choosing a thesis statement and conducting a peer review — with feedback for every correct and incorrect answer

▶ Grammar exercises

Interactive exercises on grammar, style, and punctuation — with feedback for every correct and incorrect answer

▶ Research exercises

Interactive exercises on topics such as integrating quotations, formatting in-text citations and bibliographic entries, and identifying elements needed for citing sources in MLA, APA, and CMS (*Chicago*) styles — with feedback for every correct and incorrect answer

▶ Language Debates

Brief essays by Diana Hacker that explore controversial issues of grammar and usage, such as split infinitives

▶ ESL help

Resources and strategies to help nonnative speakers improve their college writing skills

▶ Model papers

Annotated sample papers in MLA, APA, CMS (*Chicago*), and CSE styles

▶ Research and Documentation Online

Advice on finding sources and up-to-date guidelines for documenting print and online sources in MLA, APA, CMS (*Chicago*), and CSE styles

▶ Tutorials

Interactive resources that teach essential skills such as navigating *A Writer's Reference*, integrating sources, and making the most of the writing center

▶ Resources for writers and tutors

Handouts, revision checklists, and tips for visiting the writing center

▶ Additional resources

Print-format exercises for practice and links to additional online resources

Tutorials

The following tutorials will give you practice using the book's menus, index, glossary of usage, and MLA directory. Answers to the tutorials begin on page xv.

TUTORIAL 1
Using the menus

Each of the following "rules" violates the principle it expresses. Using the brief menu inside the front cover or the detailed menu inside the back cover, find the section in *A Writer's Reference* that explains the principle. Then fix the problem. Examples:

▶ *Tutors in*
~~In~~ the writing center/ ~~they~~ say that vague pronoun reference
^
is unacceptable. *G3-b*

come
▶ Be alert for irregular verbs that have ~~came~~ to you in the
^
wrong form. *G2-a*

1. A verb have to agree with its subject.
2. Each pronoun should agree with their antecedent.
3. About sentence fragments. You should avoid them.
4. Its important to use apostrophe's correctly.
5. Check for *-ed* verb endings that have been drop.
6. Discriminate careful between adjectives and adverbs.
7. If your sentence begins with a long introductory word group use a comma to separate the word group from the rest of the sentence.
8. Don't write a run-on sentence, you must connect independent clauses with a comma and a coordinating conjunction or with a semicolon.
9. A writer must be careful not to shift your point of view.
10. When dangling, watch your modifiers.

TUTORIAL 2
Using the index

Assume that you have written the following sentences and want to know the answers to the questions in brackets. Use the index at the back of the book to locate the information you need, and edit the sentences if necessary.

1. Each of the candidates have decided to participate in tonight's debate. [Should the verb be *has* or *have* to agree with *Each*?]
2. We had intended to go surfing but spent most of our vacation lying on the beach. [Should I use *lying* or *laying*?]
3. We only looked at two houses before buying the house of our dreams. [Is *only* in the right place?]
4. In Saudi Arabia it is considered ill mannered for you to accept a gift. [Is it okay to use *you* to mean "anyone in general"?]
5. In Canada, Joanne picked up several bottles of maple syrup for her sister and me. [Should I write *for her sister and I*?]

TUTORIAL 3
Using the menu system or the index

Imagine that you are in the following situations. Using either the menus or the index, find the information you need.

1. You are Ray Farley, a community college student who has been out of high school for ten years. You recall learning to put a comma between all items in a series except the last two. But you have noticed that most writers use a comma between all items. You're curious about the current rule. Which section of *A Writer's Reference* will you consult?

2. You are Maria Sanchez, a peer tutor in your university's writing center. Mike Lee, a nonnative speaker of English, has come to you for help. He is working on a rough draft that contains a number of problems with articles (*a, an,* and *the*). You know how to use articles, but you aren't able to explain the complicated rules on their correct use. Which section of *A Writer's Reference* will you and Mike Lee consult?

3. You are John Pell, engaged to marry Sophia Ju. In a note to Sophia's parents, you have written, "Thank you for giving Sophia and myself such a generous contribution toward our honeymoon." You wonder if you should write "Sophia and I" or "Sophia and me." What does *A Writer's Reference* say?

4. You are Selena Young, an intern supervisor at a housing agency. Two of your interns, Jake Gilliam and Aisha Greene, have writing problems involving -*s* endings on verbs. Jake tends to drop -*s* endings; Aisha tends to add them where they don't belong. You suspect that both problems stem from non-standard dialects spoken at home.

    Aisha and Jake are in danger of losing their jobs because your boss thinks that anyone who writes "the tenant refuse" or "the landlords agrees" is beyond hope. You disagree. Aisha and Jake have asked for your help. Where in *A Writer's Reference* can they find the rules they need?

5. You are Owen Thompson, a first-year college student. Your friend Samantha, who has completed two years of college, seems to enjoy correcting your English. Just yesterday she corrected your sentence "I felt badly about her death" to "I felt bad about her death." You're sure you've heard many educated people, including professors, say "I felt badly." Upon consulting *A Writer's Reference*, what do you discover?

TUTORIAL 4
Using the glossary of usage

Consult the glossary of usage (section W1) to see if the italicized words are used correctly. Then edit any sentences containing incorrect usage. If a sentence is correct, write "correct" after it. Example:

>   *an*
> ► The pediatrician gave my daughter ~~a~~ injection for her allergy.

1. Changing attitudes *toward* alcohol have *effected* the beer industry.
2. It is *mankind's* nature to think wisely and act foolishly.
3. This afternoon I plan to *lie* in my hammock and read.
4. Our goal this year is to *grow* our profits by 9 percent.
5. Most sleds are pulled by no *less* than two dogs and no more than ten.

TUTORIAL 5
Using the directory to MLA works cited models

Assume that you have written a short research essay on the origins of hip-hop music. You have cited the following sources in your essay, using MLA documentation, and you are ready to type your list of works cited. Turn to page 379 and use the MLA directory to locate the appropriate models. Then write a correct entry for each source and arrange the entries in a properly formatted list of works cited.

A book by Jeff Chang titled *Can't Stop, Won't Stop: A History of the Hip-Hop Generation.* The book was published in New York by St. Martin's Press in 2005.

An online article by Kay Randall called "Studying a Hip-Hop Nation." The article appeared on the University of Texas at Austin Web site, which you accessed on April 13, 2006. The last update was April 11, 2005, and the URL is <http://www.utexas.edu/features/archive/2003/hiphop.html>.

A journal article by H. Samy Alim titled "360 Degreez of Black Art Comin at You: Sista Sonia Sanchez and the Dimensions of a Black Arts Continuum." The article appears in the journal *BMa: The Sonia Sanchez Literary Review*, which is paginated by issue. The article appears on pages 15–33. The volume number is 6, the issue number is 1, and the year is 2000.

A sound recording entitled "Rapper's Delight" performed by the Sugarhill Gang on the LP *The Sugarhill Gang.* The album was released in 1979 by Sugarhill Records.

A magazine article accessed through the *InfoTrac* database *Expanded Academic ASAP*. The article, "The Roots Redefine Hip-Hop's Past," was written by Kimberly Davis and published in *Ebony* magazine in June 2003. The article appears on pages 162–64. You found this article at the Ray Cosgrove Library at Truman College in Chicago on April 13, 2006, using the URL <http://infotrac.galegroup.com>.

Answers to Tutorial 1

1. A verb has to agree with its subject. (G1-a)
2. Each pronoun should agree with its antecedent. (G3-a)
3. Avoid sentence fragments. (G5)
4. It's important to use apostrophes correctly. (P5-c and P5-e)
5. Check for *-ed* verb endings that have been dropped. (G2-d)
6. Discriminate carefully between adjectives and adverbs. (G4)
7. If your sentence begins with a long introductory word group, use a comma to separate the word group from the rest of the sentence. (P1-b)

8. Don't write a run-on sentence; you must connect independent clauses with a comma and a coordinating conjunction or with a semicolon. (G6)
9. A writer must be careful not to shift his or her [*not* their] point of view. *Or* Writers must be careful not to shift their point of view. (S4-a)
10. Watch out for dangling modifiers. (S3-e)

Answers to Tutorial 2

1. The index entry "*each*" mentions that the word is singular, so you might not need to look further to realize that the verb should be *has,* not *have.* The first page reference takes you to the entry for *each* in the glossary of usage, which directs you to G1-e and G3-a for details about why *has* is correct. The index entry "*has* vs. *have*" leads you to the chart in G1-a.
2. The index entry "*lying* vs. *laying*" takes you to section G2-b, where you will learn that *lying* (meaning "reclining or resting on a surface") is correct.
3. Look up "*only,* placement of" and you will be directed to section S3-a, which explains that limiting modifiers such as *only* should be placed before the words they modify. The sentence should read *We looked at only two houses before buying the house of our dreams.*
4. Looking up "*you,* inappropriate use of" leads you to the glossary of usage (W1) and section G3-b, which explain that *you* should not be used to mean "anyone in general." You can revise the sentence by using *a person* or *one* instead of *you,* or you can restructure the sentence completely: *In Saudi Arabia, accepting a gift is considered ill mannered.*
5. The index entries "*I* vs. *me*" and "*me* vs. *I*" take you to section G3-c, which explains why *me* is correct.

Answers to Tutorial 3

1. Section P1-c states that, although usage varies, most experts advise using a comma between all items in a series — to prevent possible misreadings or ambiguities. To find this section, Ray Farley would probably use the menu system.
2. Maria Sanchez and Mike Lee would consult section E3, on articles. This section is easy to locate in the menu system.
3. Section G3-c explains why *Sophia and me* is correct. To find section G3-c, John Pell could use the menu system if he knew to look under "Problems with pronouns." Otherwise, he could look up "*I* vs. *me*" in the index. Pell could also look up "*myself*" in the index or he could consult the glossary of usage (W1), where a cross-reference would direct him to section G3-c.
4. Selena Young's interns could turn to sections G1 and G2-c for help. Young could use the menu system to find these sections if she knew to look under "Subject-verb agreement" or "Standard English verb forms." If she wasn't sure about the grammatical terminology, she could look up "*-s,* as verb ending" or "Verbs, *-s* form of" in the index.
5. Section G4-b explains why *I felt bad about her death* is correct. To find section G4-b, Owen Thompson could use the menu system if he knew that *bad* versus *badly* is a choice between an adjective and an adverb. Otherwise he could look up "*bad, badly*" in the index or the glossary of usage (W1).

Answers to Tutorial 4

1. Changing attitudes toward alcohol have *affected* the beer industry.
2. It is *human* nature to think wisely and act foolishly.
3. Correct
4. Our goal this year is to *increase* our profits by 9 percent.
5. Most sleds are pulled by no *fewer* than two dogs and no more than ten.

Answers to Tutorial 5

Alim, H. Samy. "360 Degreez of Black Art Comin at You: Sista Sonia Sanchez and the Dimensions of a Black Arts Continuum." BMa: The Sonia Sanchez Literary Review 6.1 (2000): 15-33.

Chang, Jeff. Can't Stop, Won't Stop: A History of the Hip-Hop Generation. New York: St. Martin's, 2005.

Davis, Kimberly. "The Roots Redefine Hip-Hop's Past." Ebony June 2003: 162-64. Expanded Academic ASAP. InfoTrac. Ray Cosgrove Lib., Truman Coll., Chicago. 13 Apr. 2006 <http://infotrac.galegroup.com>.

Randall, Kay. "Studying a Hip-Hop Nation." University of Texas at Austin. 11 Apr. 2005. 13 Apr. 2006 <http://www.utexas.edu/features/archives/2003/hiphop.html>.

Sugarhill Gang. "Rapper's Delight." The Sugarhill Gang. LP. Sugarhill, 1979.

Preface for instructors

Publisher's note

> When Bedford and I invented the quick-reference format — with
> its main menu, tabbed dividers, and lie-flat binding — . . . we had
> no idea that *A Writer's Reference* would become so popular (or so
> widely imitated). My goals were more modest. I hoped that the for-
> mat and the title would send a clear message: *A Writer's Reference*
> is meant to be consulted as needed; it is not a set of grammar
> lessons to be studied in a vacuum. . . . Instructors across the coun-
> try tell me that their students can and do use the book on their
> own, keeping it flipped open next to their computers.
>
> > Diana Hacker (1942–2004),
> > from the Preface for Instructors,
> > *A Writer's Reference,* Fifth Edition

In her trademark lucid style, Diana Hacker describes making publishing history. *A Writer's Reference* is not only the most widely
adopted English handbook on the market but also the best-selling
college textbook of any kind in any discipline. It literally revolution-
ized the handbook genre. Users of the book routinely tell us that
A Writer's Reference is the easiest handbook to use — a book that
helps students find what they need and understand what they find.

Like all of the innovations that Diana Hacker brought to the
genre of handbooks, the innovations of *A Writer's Reference* came
from her teaching. She was able to take everything she knew from
her thirty-five years of teaching and put it to work on every page of
her books. Diana carefully observed how students actually used
handbooks — mainly as references — and designed a book that
would work better for them. The tabbed dividers and comb binding,
which allow *A Writer's Reference* to lie open on any page, make it
easier for students to find the information they need as quickly as

possible. Once they get to the right page, the information is easy for them to understand on their own. The book's patient, respectful tone; its clear, concise explanations; and its hand-edited examples give students the help they need. Even though many other handbooks have imitated the format, no one understands as Diana did how format and content have to work together to make a truly useful handbook.

Although the first edition grew primarily out of Diana Hacker's own teaching experiences, subsequent editions reflect the experiences of the thousands of instructors using the books in their classrooms and of the millions of students who have found it helpful. For this new edition, we relied on advice from an extraordinary group of reviewers who kept reminding us what their students need. More than five hundred dedicated and experienced composition instructors reviewed the sixth edition. More than thirty of them served as an editorial advisory board; they read and commented on every word of this edition, making sure that it will work as well for their students as it always has and that the new material meets the high standards of a Hacker handbook.

With her team of Bedford editors, Diana had mapped out a plan for the sixth edition. Based on this plan, a talented group of contributing authors revised this edition, putting themselves at the service of the book while bringing their own classroom experience to everything they did. Nancy Sommers, Tom Jehn, and Jane Rosenzweig — all of whom teach in the Harvard Expository Writing Program — helped revise the coverage of the writing process and research. Marcy Carbajal Van Horn, teacher of composition and ESL at Santa Fe Community College (FL), revised the ESL coverage. Diana was a huge fan of Nancy Sommers's work because it focused on student writing, drawing on Nancy's teaching at the University of Oklahoma and Rutgers as well as at Harvard. Diana was eager to have insights from Nancy's recent longitudinal study of student writing in the book. Tom Jehn is the clear and patient writing teacher that Diana always was, especially in helping students work with sources. Jane Rosenzweig is the skilled writer Diana always hoped for in a coauthor. Marcy Carbajal Van Horn creates practical and accessible content for a broad range of students — starting with her own — as Diana always did.

A Writer's Reference has always been a team effort between Diana and her editors at Bedford/St. Martin's, and that team is still in place. I was Diana's editor on the first edition of every one of her handbooks, including *A Writer's Reference*, and have been a part of every book since. Special thanks go to Chuck Christensen for understanding what makes a great handbook author and for knowing he had found one in Diana Hacker. At the heart of the Hacker team is Diana's longtime editor, executive editor Michelle Clark, the most skilled, creative editor we could wish for. Development editors Ellen Kuhl and Michelle McSweeney, veterans of many Hacker handbooks, made sure that every word in this book sounds like Diana's voice. Claire Seng-Niemoeller has designed every Hacker handbook since the first and has again retained the clean, uncluttered look of the book while making more use of color. Having copyedited every Hacker handbook, Barbara Flanagan has been hearing Diana's voice for more than twenty years. Diana credited her with the clarity and consistency that is a Hacker hallmark. Senior production editor Anne Noonan kept us all on track with her persistence, sharp eye, and concern for every detail. Assistant production editor Amy Derjue provided detailed assistance throughout the page proof review. Editor in chief Karen Henry and managing editor Elizabeth Schaaf have worked on these books from the beginning and remain committed to Diana's vision. New media editors Mara Weible and Amy Hurd Gershman expanded the new media offerings, making them as easy to use as the book itself. Stellar editorial assistant Jennifer Lyford managed various projects and made sure that we heard from as many users as possible. We all remain committed to maintaining the high level of quality of Hacker handbooks.

The result is a revision that does what *A Writer's Reference* has always done: It works. Our hope is that students will keep flipping it open to find the best answers to their questions about writing.

Joan Feinberg
President, Bedford/St. Martin's

Features of the sixth edition

What's new

NEW VISUALS THAT TEACH CITATION AT A GLANCE.   New full-color, annotated facsimiles of original sources show students where to look for publication information in a book, a periodical, a Web site, and a source accessed in a database. These visuals help students find the information they need to cite print and online materials accurately and responsibly.

ADVICE THAT HELPS STUDENTS MAINTAIN THEIR VOICE WHILE WRITING FROM SOURCES.   Thoroughly revised coverage of integrating sources teaches students how to go beyond patchwork research writing.

Section MLA-3 shows students how to lead into — and get out of — sources while keeping the source material in context and maintaining their own line of argument.

GUIDELINES THAT HELP STUDENTS UNDERSTAND HOW SOURCES CAN FUNCTION IN THEIR WRITING. A new section (MLA-1c) teaches students to consider the varying roles that sources can play in research writing.

NEW CHARTS THAT OFFER PRACTICAL ADVICE FOR USING SOURCES. New quick-reference charts on determining whether a source is "scholarly," on selecting appropriate versions of electronic sources, and on avoiding Internet plagiarism help students meet the challenges of research writing in the digital age.

A NEW EMPHASIS ON ACADEMIC WRITING. A new tabbed section (A) equips students with strategies for writing well in any college course; it brings new chapters on writing about texts and writing in the disciplines together with a revised chapter on argument.

GUIDELINES FOR WRITING ABOUT VERBAL AND VISUAL TEXTS. A new section (A1) provides advice and models for annotating, outlining, summarizing, and analyzing both verbal texts (such as essays and articles) and visual texts (such as advertisements and photographs).

A NEW CHAPTER ON WRITING IN THE DISCIPLINES. *A Writer's Reference* offers more help for students as they write in courses outside of the humanities. It explains the common features of all good college writing and provides practical advice for approaching writing assignments in all disciplines.

MORE HELP WITH WRITING ARGUMENTS. Revised coverage of counterargument teaches students how to strengthen their writing by anticipating and responding to objections.

NEW QUICK-ACCESS CHARTS. The sixth edition features new charts that help writers navigate common writing challenges: understanding a writing assignment, making use of advice from peer reviewers, writing a conclusion, reading actively, and analyzing visuals.

MEETS THE NEEDS OF A BROADER RANGE OF ESL STUDENTS. Thoroughly revised ESL coverage considers the experiences of college students who may be proficient English speakers but who continue to struggle with writing well in English.

MORE HELP FOR THE MOST TROUBLESOME SENTENCE-LEVEL PROBLEMS.
Developed with the help of ESL specialists, the sixth edition offers
stronger support for using verbs, articles, and prepositions correctly. New charts offer at-a-glance help for nonnative speakers of
English.

**CRUCIAL ADVICE ON ACADEMIC CONVENTIONS — FOR NATIVE AS WELL AS
NONNATIVE SPEAKERS.**   New boxed tips teach *academic English* —
or how to go about writing well at an American college. Throughout
the book, these nuggets of advice — on topics such as plagiarism,
writing arguments, and understanding writing assignments — help
students meet college expectations.

AN UNCLUTTERED PAGE DESIGN.   The book's new, more colorful design
presents complex material and new visual elements as simply as
possible. Because grammar rules and hand-edited examples are
highlighted in color, students can easily skim the book's central sections for quick answers to questions. Charts and boxes are easy to
find and, just as important, easy to skip.

NEW SAMPLE PAPERS.   Four new major papers show good writing
and proper formatting: an argument essay; an analysis of an article; an MLA-style research essay; and an APA-style review of the
literature.

UPDATED GRAMMAR CHECKER BOXES.   A Diana Hacker innovation,
the fifty grammar checker boxes have been updated to reflect the
way current grammar and spell checker programs work. Students
will read helpful advice about the capabilities and limitations of
these programs.

FLEXIBLE CONTENT THAT HELPS YOU MEET THE NEEDS OF YOUR STUDENTS.
Supplemental content for ESL, writing in the disciplines, visual
rhetoric, and writing about literature is available for packaging or
for custom publishing to create a handbook that supports your
course. In addition, a version of *A Writer's Reference* with integrated
exercises will be available in 2007.

What's the same

We have kept the features that have made *A Writer's Reference*
work so well for so many students and instructors. These features,
detailed here, will be familiar to users of the previous edition.

COLOR-CODED MAIN MENU AND TABBED DIVIDERS. The main menu directs students to orange, blue, green, and white tabbed dividers; the color coding makes it easy for students to identify and flip to the section they need. The documentation sections are further color-coded: blue for MLA, green for APA, and brown for CMS.

USER-FRIENDLY INDEX. This index, which Diana Hacker wrote herself and which was carefully updated for this edition, helps students find what they are looking for even if they don't know grammatical terminology. When facing a choice between *I* and *me*, for example, students may not know to look up "Case" or even "Pronoun, case of." They are more likely to look up "*I*" or "*me*," so the index includes entries for "*I* vs. *me*" and "*me* vs. *I*." Similar user-friendly entries appear throughout the index.

Index entries include the letter of the tabbed section before the page number of the indexed term (**G**: 192). Users can flip directly to the correct tabbed divider, such as G (for Grammatical sentences) before tracking down the page number.

QUICK-REFERENCE CHARTS. Many of the handbook's charts help students review for common problems in their own writing, such as fragments and subject-verb agreement. Other charts summarize important material: a checklist for global revision, strategies for avoiding sexist language, guidelines for evaluating Web sites, and so on.

DISCIPLINE-SPECIFIC RHETORICAL ADVICE FOR MLA, APA, AND CMS (*CHICAGO*) STYLES. Advice on drafting a thesis, avoiding plagiarism, and integrating sources is illustrated for all three major documentation styles — MLA, APA, and CMS (*Chicago*) — in three color-coded sections. Examples are related to topics appropriate to the disciplines that typically use each style: English and other humanities (MLA), social sciences (APA), and history (CMS).

What's on the companion Web site
<http://dianahacker.com/writersref>

RESOURCES FOR WRITERS AND TUTORS. New writing center resources on the companion Web site offer help for both tutors and writers: checklists for responding to a wide array of assignments, tips for preparing for a visit to the writing center, hints for making the best use of advice from tutors, and helpsheets for common writing problems — the same kinds of handouts students see in the writing center — all available in printable format.

ELECTRONIC GRAMMAR EXERCISES.   For online practice, students can access more than one thousand exercise items — on every topic in the handbook — with feedback written by Diana Hacker. Most of the exercises are scorable. Exercises that call for editing are labeled "edit and compare." They ask students to edit sentences and compare their versions with possible revisions.

ELECTRONIC RESEARCH AND WRITING EXERCISES.   Scorable electronic exercises on matters such as avoiding plagiarism, integrating sources, documenting sources, and identifying citation elements give students ample practice with these critical topics. Scorable exercises on thesis statements, peer review, point of view, transitions, and other writing topics support students throughout the composing process.

LANGUAGE DEBATES.   To encourage students to think about the rationales for a rule and then make their own rhetorical decisions, Diana Hacker wrote twenty brief essays that explore controversial issues of grammar and usage, such as split infinitives and *who* versus *whom*. The Web site for the sixth edition features two additional debates written by style expert Barbara Wallraff.

MODEL PAPERS.   Model papers for MLA, APA, CMS (*Chicago*), and CSE styles illustrate both the design and the content of researched writing. Annotations highlight key points about each paper's style, content, and documentation.

RESEARCH AND DOCUMENTATION ONLINE.   This online resource helps students conduct research and document their sources. Reference librarian Barbara Fister has updated her advice on finding sources and has provided new links to resources in a variety of disciplines; she continues to maintain the research portion of the site. Guidelines for documenting print and online sources in MLA, APA, CMS (*Chicago*), and CSE styles are also kept up-to-date.

EXTRA HELP FOR ESL WRITERS.   For native and nonnative speakers alike, this area of the site offers advice and strategies for understanding college expectations and for writing well on college assignments. Authored by Marcy Carbajal Van Horn (assistant professor of English and ESL at Santa Fe Community College, FL), it includes many helpful charts, exercises and activities, advice for working with sources, and an annotated student essay.

ACCESS TO AN ONLINE E-HANDBOOK. With the purchase of a print version of the handbook, students also have premium access to an electronic version of *A Writer's Reference*, conveniently located at the companion site.

THE INSTRUCTOR SITE. Accessible from the student site, this password-protected Web site offers additional resources such as diagnostic tests and tutorials and serves as a portal for retrieving student exercise results.

Ancillaries for students

PRINT RESOURCES

Exercises to Accompany A WRITER'S REFERENCE (with answer key)

Developmental Exercises to Accompany A WRITER'S REFERENCE (with answer key)

Working with Sources: Exercises to Accompany A WRITER'S REFERENCE (with answer key)

Research and Documentation in the Electronic Age, Fourth Edition

Language Debates, Second Edition

Writing about Literature

Extra Help for ESL Writers

Writing in the Disciplines: Advice and Models

ONLINE RESOURCES

A Writer's Reference companion Web site (See the On the Web box on p. xi.)

Comment with *A Writer's Reference*

Ancillaries for instructors

PROFESSIONAL RESOURCES FOR INSTRUCTORS

Teaching Composition: Background Readings

The Bedford Guide for Writing Tutors, Fourth Edition

The Bedford Bibliography for Teachers of Writing, Sixth Edition

ONLINE RESOURCES FOR INSTRUCTORS

A Writer's Reference instructor site at <http://dianahacker.com/writersref>

Exercise Masters, print-format versions of all the exercises in the book

Quiz Masters, print-format quizzes on key topics in the book

Electronic Diagnostic Tests, a test bank for instructors' use

Transparency Masters, useful charts, examples, and visuals from the book

Preparing for the CLAST

Preparing for the THEA

In addition, all of the resources within *Re:Writing* <http://bedfordstmartins.com/rewriting> are available for free to users of *A Writer's Reference*. Resources include tutorials, exercises, diagnostics, technology help, and model documents — all written by our most widely adopted authors.

Other composition resources by Bedford/St. Martin's

The following resources are available for packaging with *A Writer's Reference*:

ix visual exercises (CD-ROM), Cheryl E. Gall and Kristin L. Arola. Introduces the fundamentals of visual composition in an interactive medium

i·cite visualizing sources (CD-ROM), Doug Downs. Introduces students to how sources work and provides interactive practice

i·claim visualizing argument (CD-ROM), Patrick Clauss. Introduces argument concepts with a range of multimedia examples; includes assignments

Oral Presentations in the Composition Course: A Brief Guide, Matthew Duncan and Gustav W. Friedrich

For a complete list, contact your sales representative or visit <http://bedfordstmartins.com/composition>.

Course management content

A variety of student and instructor resources developed for *A Writer's Reference* are ready for use in course management systems.

Acknowledgments

Diana Hacker worked with us to map out her goals for the sixth edition. We called on a number of experienced, creative individuals to develop the sixth edition with Diana's plan as the foundation.

Contributing authors

The contributors brought both expertise and enthusiasm to the project. They drafted new content and rethought existing content to make certain that *A Writer's Reference* reaches a broader range of students and meets their varied needs.

> **Nancy Sommers**, Sosland Director of Expository Writing at Harvard University, has also taught composition at Rutgers University and at Monmouth College and has directed the writing program at the University of Oklahoma. A two-time Braddock Award winner, Sommers is well known for her research and publications on student writing. Her articles "Revision Strategies of Student and Experienced Writers" and "Responding to Student Writing" are two of the most widely read in the field. Her recent work involves a longitudinal study of undergraduate writing.

> **Tom Jehn** teaches composition and directs the writing across the disciplines program at Harvard University. A recipient of numerous teaching awards both at Harvard and at the University of Virginia, he also leads professional development seminars on writing instruction for public high school teachers through the Calderwood Writing Fellows Project.

> **Jane Rosenzweig**, a published author of fiction and nonfiction, teaches composition and directs the writing center at Harvard University. She has also taught writing at Yale University and the University of Iowa.

> **Marcy Carbajal Van Horn**, assistant professor of English and ESL at Santa Fe Community College (FL), teaches composition to native and nonnative speakers of English and teaches the advanced ESL writing course. She has also taught university-level academic writing and critical thinking at Instituto Tecnológico y de Estudios Superiores in Mexico.

Editorial Advisory Board

We asked a number of longtime users of the book and several nonusers to serve as editorial advisers. They looked carefully at all new and substantially revised sections of the sixth edition to make certain that the book is still as effective as it has always been in their classrooms. We thank them for their thoughtful and candid reviews.

Joanne Addison, University of Colorado, Denver

Derick Burleson, University of Alaska, Fairbanks

Paige Byam, Northern Kentucky University

Elizabeth Canfield, Virginia Commonwealth University

Richard Carr, University of Alaska, Fairbanks

Michele Cheung, University of Southern Maine, Portland

Jon Cullick, Northern Kentucky University

David Endicott, Tacoma Community College (WA)

Lin Fraser, Sacramento City College (CA)

Hank Galmish, Green River Community College (WA)

Nancy Gish, University of Southern Maine, Portland

Jacqueline Gray, St. Charles Community College (MO)

Barclay Green, Northern Kentucky University

Karen Grossweiner, University of Alaska, Fairbanks

D. J. Henry, Daytona Beach Community College

Kandace Knudson, Sacramento City College (CA)

Tonya Krouse, Northern Kentucky University

Tamara Kuzmenkov, Tacoma Community College (WA)

Cheryl Laz, University of Southern Maine, Portland

Lydia Lynn Lewellen, Tacoma Community College (WA)

Jeanette Lonia, Delaware Technical and Community College

Walter Lowe, Green River Community College (WA)

Michael Mackey, Community College of Denver (CO)

Tammy Mata, Tarrant County College (TX)

Holly McSpadden, Missouri Southern State University

Liora Moriel, University of Maryland, College Park

Patricia Murphy, Missouri Southern State University

Melissa Nicolas, University of Louisiana, Lafayette

Diane Allen O'Heron, Broome Community College (NY)

Sarah Quirk, Waubonsee Community College (IL)

Ann Smith, Modesto Junior College (CA)

Steve Thomas, Community College of Denver (CO)

Nick Tingle, University of California, Santa Barbara

Terry Myers Zawacki, George Mason University (VA)

Reviewers

For their many helpful suggestions, we would like to thank a perceptive group of reviewers. Some answered a detailed questionnaire about the fifth edition; others reviewed manuscript for the sixth edition.

Barry Abrams, Sierra College (CA); Melanie Abrams, California State University, San Bernardino; Susan Achziger, Community College of Aurora (CO); Jo Acres-Devine, University of Alaska, Southeast; D. Michelle Adkerson, Nashville State Technical Community College (TN); Judy Andree, University of Alaska, Southeast; Rebecca Argall, University of Memphis (TN); Marianne Arieux, Empire State College (NY); Diann Arinder, Jackson Preparatory School (MS); Janice Aslanian, Hope College (MI); Greg Barnhisel, Duquesne University (PA); Dana Basinger, Samford University (AL); Dennis Beach, Saint John's University (MN); Diana Bell, University of Alabama, Huntsville; Sally Bell, University of Montevallo (AL); Barbara Bengels, Hofstra University (NY); Rick Beno, Padua Academy (DE); Cameron Bentley, Augusta Technical Institute (GA); Mary Bettley, Lesley University (MA); Nilanjana Bhattacharjya, Cornell University (NY); Desha Bierbaum, Lesley University (MA); Cynthia Bily, Adrian College (MI); Delmar Bishop, Pomona High School (CO); Shalom Black, Catholic University of America (DC); Keva Boone, Barry University (FL); Robin Bott, Adrian College (MI); Kimberly Bovee, Tidewater Community College (VA); Martha Bowden, Kennesaw State (GA); Brad Bowers, Barry University (FL); Mary Boyes, Tusculum College (TN); Molly Boyle, Massachusetts Bay Community College; Karla Braig, Loras College (IA); Angela Branch, John Tyler Community College (VA); Jennifer Brezina, College of the Canyons (CA); Kristi Brock, Northern Kentucky University; Angier Brock Caudle, Virginia Commonwealth University; Elaine Brooks, CUNY Brooklyn College (NY); Barry Brown, Missouri Southern State University; Cheryl Brown, Towson University (MD); Laura Brown, Central Alabama Community College; Shanti Bruce, Indiana University of Pennsylvania; Richard Bullock, Wright State University (OH); William Burgos, Long Island University, Brooklyn (NY); Richard Burke, Lynchburg College (VA); Charles Burm, Monroe Community College (NY); Ellen Butki, University of Texas at Austin; Barb Butler, Bellevue Community College (WA); Candace Byrne, Shasta College (CA); Stephen Calatrello, Calhoun State Community College (AL); Linda Caldwell, Towson University (MD); Catherine Calloway, Arkansas State University, Main Campus; Jorinde Canden Berg, Montgomery College, Germantown (MD); Phyllis Carey, Mount Mary College (WI); Cheryl Carpinello, Alameda Senior High School (CO); Pat Cearley, South Plains College (TX); Sherry Chapman, Modesto Junior College (CA); Nishi Chawla, University of Maryland University College; Marjorie Childers, Elms College (MA); Angela Christman, Loyola College (MD); Greg Clark, Brigham Young University (UT); Anne Clark, St. Cloud State University (MN); Gladys Cleland, SUNY Morrisville (NY); Joanne Clements, University of Rochester Medical School (NY); Cheryl Cobb, Tidewater Community College (VA); Jill Coe, Southwest Texas Junior College; Tammy Conard-Salvo, Purdue University (IA); Magana Conception, Garden City Community College (KS); Linda Conra, Curry College (MA); Trish Conrad, Hutchinson Community College (KS); Linda Conway, Howard College (TX); Cheryl Corbiell, Maui Community College (HI); Jennifer Courtney-Pooler, University of North Carolina, Charlotte; Julie Cox, University of California, Santa Cruz; Michelle Cox, University of New Hampshire; Donna Craine, Front Range Community College/Westminster (CO); Delmas Crisp, Wesleyan College (GA); Beth Crookston, Stark State College of Technology (OH); Pam Cross, Stockton State College (NJ); Eileen Crowe, University of North Carolina, Asheville; Debbie Cunningham, Adams State College (CO); Stephen Curley, Texas A&M, Galveston; Billye Currie, Samford University (AL); Sarah Curtis, Consumnes River College (CA); Christopher Dainele, Massachusetts Bay Community College; Helen Dale, University of Wisconsin, Eau Claire; Sarah Dangelantonio, Franklin Pierce College (NH); Cynthia Davidson, SUNY Stony Brook (NY); Matthew Davis, University of Puget Sound (WA); Sister Mary Davlin, Dominican University (IL); Mary De Nys, George Mason University (VA); Ann Dean, University of Southern Maine, Portland; Deborah Dean, Brigham Young University (UT); Renee Dechert, Northwest College (WY); Jeffrey Decker, University of California, Los Angeles; Margie Dernaika, Southwest Tennessee Community College; Kathryn De Zur, SUNY Delhi (NY); Kristen di Gennaro, Pace University (NY); Theresa Dolan, Los Angeles Trade Technical College (CA); Lynn Domina, SUNY Delhi (NY); Patricia Don, San Jose State University (CA); Cecilia Donohue, Madonna University (MI); Tony D'Souza, Shasta College (CA); Deb Dusek, North Dakota State College of Science; Chitralekha Duttagupta, Arizona State University; Scott Earle, Tacoma Community College (WA); Marie Eckstrom, Rio Hondo College (CA); Martha Edmonds, University of Richmond (VA); Richard Eichman, Sauk Valley Community College (IL); Mary Ellen, University of North Carolina, Charlotte; Lynette Emanuel, Wisconsin Indianhead Technical Institute; Charlene Engleking, Lindenwood University (MO); Bill Eppright, Northwestern College (MN); Douglas Eyman, Michigan State University; Deanna Fassett, San Jose State University (CA); Deborah Fleming, Ashland University (OH); John Fleming, De Anza College (CA); Maryann Fleming-McCall, Atlantic Cape Community College (NJ); Jessica Fordham Kidd, University of Alabama; P. Forson-Williams, McDaniel College (MD); Deanna Foster, Lassen College (CA); Bonnie Fox, D'Youville College (NY); Catherine Fraga, California State University, Sacramento; Martha Francescato, George Mason University (VA); Michael Frank, Bentley College (MA); Traci Freeman, University of Colorado, Colorado Springs; Christina French, Diablo Valley College (CA); Steve Frogge, Missouri Western State University; Jacqueline Fulmer, University of California, Berkeley; Karen Gardiner, University of Alabama; Wayne Garrett, Lipscomb University (TN); Susan Garrett, McDaniel College (MD); Steven

Gehring, SUNY Stony Brook (NY); Dennis Geisler, Columbia College (MO); Gina Genova, University of California, Santa Barbara; James Gifford, Mohawk Valley Community College (NY); Jane Gilligan, Assumption College (MA); Susan Gimprich, Fairleigh Dickinson University (NJ); Tracey Glaessgen, Southwest Missouri State University; Norman Golar, University of Alabama; Bertrand Goldgar, Lawrence University (WI); Amy Goodwin, Randolph-Macon College (VA); Ricia Gordon, Landmark College (VT); Rebecca Gorman, Metropolitan State College of Denver (CO); William Gorski, West Los Angeles College (CA); Susan Gorsky, University of California, Santa Cruz; Gwen Gray Schwartz, University of Arizona; Robert Greenwald, Dominican University (IL); Katie Guest, University of North Carolina, Greensboro; Max Guggenhiemer, Lynchburg College (VA); Diana Gyler, Azusa Pacific University (CA); Joan Haahr, Yeshiva University (NY); Thomas Hackett, CUNY Brooklyn College (NY); Michelle Halbach, Widener University (DE); Susan Halio, Long Island University, Brooklyn (NY); Peggy Hamilton, San Joaquin Delta College (CA); Robin Hammerman, Stevens Institute of Technology (NJ); Kathleen Hammond, Brookdale Community College (NJ); Jefferson Hancock, Cabrillo College (CA); Heidi Hanrahan, University of North Carolina, Greensboro; Katie Hanson, Augustana College (IL); John Hanvey, Barry University (FL); Lisa Harbo, University of Alaska, Fairbanks; Gloria Hardy, Saint John's University (MN); Eunice Hargett, Broward Community College, Central (FL); Mitchell Harris, University of Texas; Terese Hartman, Lynchburg College (VA); Kip Hartvigsen, Brigham Young University, Idaho; Lisa Hastings, Delaware Technical and Community College; Gary Hatch, Brigham Young University (UT); Nancy Hayward, Indiana University of Pennsylvania; Shelly Hedstrom, Palm Beach Community College (FL); Ruth Heller, Eastern Connecticut State University; Diane Henningfeld, Adrian College (MI); Bridgette Henry, University of Missouri, Kansas City; Patricia Henshaw, Sacramento City College (CA); Leah Herman, Pitzer College (CA); Kathleen Hickey, Dominican University (NY); Sharon Hileman, Sul Ross State University (TX); Cheryl Hill, Nova Southeastern University (FL); Vicki Hill, Brewton-Parker College (GA); Lisa Hodgens, Piedmont College (GA); Kathleen Hoffman, Cambridge Community College (MN); John Hogwood, Wayland Baptist University (TX); Deborah Holler, Empire State College (NY); Camille Lee Hornbeck, Tarrant County Community College (TX); Alice Horning, Oakland University (CA); Tai Houser, Broward Community College, North (FL); James Hunter, Gonzaga University (WA); Michael Hustedde, St. Ambrose University (IA); Marie Iglesias-Cardinale, Genessee Community College (NY); Robin Inboden, Wittenberg University (OH); Alyson Indrunas, Everett Community College (WA); James Inman, University of Tennessee, Chattanooga; Sherri Inness, Miami University, Hamilton (OH); Ginger Irwin, Colgate University (NY); James

Isbell, Santiago Canyon College (CA); Kathy Ivey, Lenoir-Rhyne College (NC); Lisa Jackson, University of North Texas; Ian Jacobs, New School University (NY); Dawnelle Jager, Syracuse University (NY); Glenda James, Calhoun State Community College (AL); Susan James, Curry College (MA); Mary Jo Stirling, Santa Monica College (CA); Carol Johnson, Virginia Wesleyan College; Sue Johnson, Sierra College (CA); Nancy Johnson Squaire, Sheridan College (WY); Jennifer Jones, University of Colorado, Boulder; Jay Jordan, Pennsylvania State University; Paul Juhasz, Tarrant County Community College (TX); Demetrios Kapetanakos, Queensborough Community College (NY); Elizabeth Katz, University of New Mexico; Janet Kay, Leeward Community College (HI); Laura Kay, John F. Kennedy University (CA); Joshua Keels, Community College of Vermont, Burlington; Elizabeth Keifer, Tunxis Community College (CT); Sue Keith, Guilford College (NC); Roberta Kelly, Washington State University; Gilda Kelsey, University of Delaware; Jan Kinch, Edinboro University of Pennsylvania; Lola King, Trinity Valley Community College (TX); Liz Kleinfeld, Red Rocks Community College (CO); Matt Kozusko, Ursinus College (PA); Carrie Krantz-Fischer, Washtenaw Community College (MI); Michelle Ladd, California State University, Los Angeles; Gina Ladinsky, Santa Monica College (CA); Lauren LaFauci, University of Michigan, Ann Arbor; John Lang, Emory and Henry College (VA); Margaret Lattimore, Gardner-Webb University (NC); Sally Lavender, Lipscomb University (TN); Joe Law, Wright State University (OH); Amy Lawlor, Pasadena City College (CA); Robert Lawrence, Jefferson Community College (KY); Kathleen Lazarus, Daytona Beach Community College (FL); Andria Leduc, Open Learning Agency (BC); Catharine Lee, Wesleyan College (GA); Michelle Lee, Minnesota State University; Kathy LeGrand, Olympic Heights High School (FL); Lindsay Lewan, Arapahoe Community College (CO); James Livingston, Northern Michigan University; Alice Longaker, University of Northern Colorado; Sonia Maasik, University of California, Los Angeles; Joan Maiers, Marylhurst University (OR); Ceil Malek, University of Colorado, Colorado Springs; Lisa Mallory, Atlanta Metropolitan College (GA); Ajuan Mance, Mills College (CA); Kate Mangelsdorf, University of Texas, El Paso; Travis Mann, Tarrant County Community College (TX); Nicole Marafioti, Cornell University (NY); Annette March, California State University, Monterey Bay; Pete Marcoux, El Camino Community College (CA); Barbara Martin, University of Cincinnati (OH); Joann Martin, Wisconsin Indianhead Technical Institute; Elizabeth Martinez, University of Connecticut; David Maruyama, Long Beach City College (CA); Pat Mathias, Itasca Community College (MN); Leanne Maunu, Palomar Community College (CA); Jennifer McCann, Bay de Noc Community College (MI); Barbara McClain, Contra Costa College (CA); Julia McGregor, Inver Hills Community College (MN); Andrea McKenzie, New York University; James McLaughlin, Master's College and Seminary (CA); Sara McLaughlin, Texas Technical University; Vicky Melograno, Atlantic Cape Community College (NJ); Agnetta Mendoza, Nashville State Technical Community College (TN); Gayle Mercer, Southwest Missouri State; Carol Messing, Northwood University (MI); Allan Metcalf, MacMurray College (IL); Donna Metcalf, Springfield College (IL); Steve Michael, Wayland Baptist University (TX); Marlene Michels, Mid Michigan Community College; Ilene Miele, University of California, Santa Barbara; David Miller, Victor Valley College (CA); Jack Miller, Normandale Community College (MN); Ruth Miller, University of Louisville (KY); Wendy Moffat, Dickinson College (PA); Scott Moncrieff, Andrews University (MI); Jayne Moneysmith, Kent State University (OH); Bryan Moore, Arkansas State University, Main Campus; Matthew Moore, Roberts Wesleyan College (NY); Robert Morace, Daemen College (NY); Dan Morgan, Scott Community College, Bettendorf (IA); Jennifer Morrison, Niagara University (NY); Gala Muench, North Idaho College (ID); Terry Muller, Cambridge College (MA); Deborah Mutnick, Long Island University, Brooklyn (NY); Linda Myers, California State University, Sacramento; Lyndall Nairn, Lynchburg College (VA); James Nash, Montclair State University (NJ); Michelle Nash, Union College (NE); Claire Nava, California State University, Fullerton; Jeffrey Nelson, University of Alabama; Stephen Newmann, Montgomery College, Germantown (MD); Corrine Nicolas, Tusculum College (TN); Jennifer Niester, Central Michigan University; Sylvia Nosworthy, Walla Walla College (WA); Catherine O'Callaghan, Community College of Vermont, Brattleboro; David Okamura-Wilson, East Carolina University (NC); Ben Opipari, Colgate College (NY); Scott Orme, Spokane Community College (WA); Christina Ortmeier-Hooper, University of New Hampshire; Mary O'Sullivan, Western Wisco Technical College (WI); Liz Parker, Nashville State Technical Community College (TN); Allison Parker, Southeastern Community College (NC); M. Elizabeth Parker, Nashville State Technical Community College (TN); Joanne Parsons, Eastern Oregon University (OR); Karen Pass, Empire State College (NY); Mary Pat, Dominican University (IL); David Paul, SUNY Morrisville (NY); Craig Payne, Indian Hills Community College (IA); Tammy Peery, Montgomery College, Germantown (MD); Myra Perry, University of North Carolina, Charlotte; Todd Petersen, Southern Utah University; Stephen Petrina, University of British Columbia; Diane Philen, Sinte Gleska University (SD); Christine Pipitone-Herron, Raritan Valley Community College (NJ); Susan Piqueira, Tunxis Community College (CT); Neil Placky, Broward Community College-South (FL); Faith Plvan, Syracuse University (NY); Robert Prescott, Bradley University (IL); Mary Lou Price, University of Texas, Austin; Ben Rafoth, Indiana University of Pennsylvania; Anniqua Rana, Canada College (CA); Vanessa Rasmussen, Rider University (NJ); Kokila Ravi, Atlanta Metropolitan College (GA);

Susan Regan, Cloud County Community College (KS); Paul Reid, Chippewa Valley Technical College (WI); Steven Reynolds, College of the Siskiyous (CA); Angela Ricciardi, Plymouth State College (NH); Clai Rice, University of Louisiana, Lafayette; Jeff Rice, Wayne State University (MI); Aaron Ritzenberg, Brandeis University (MA); Marilyn Roberts, Waynesburg College (PA); Lourdes Rodriguez-Florido, Broward Community College South (FL); Timothy Rogers, Furman University (SC); Teri Rosen, CUNY Hunter College (NY); Michelle Ross, Indiana University (IN); Deborah Rossen-Knill, University of Rochester (NY); Jennifer Rosti, Roanoke College (VA); Henry Ruminski, Wright State University (OH); Carol Russo, SUNY Stony Brook (NY); Leigh Ryan, University of Maryland; Kristen Salsbury, University of California, Irvine; Art Saltzmann, Missouri Southern State University; Mark Sanders, Three Rivers Community College (MO); Mark Sanford, Suffolk University (MA); Lilia Savova, Indiana University of Pennsylvania; Elizabeth Sawin, Missouri Western State University; Suzy Sayre, Towson University (MD); Bret Scaliter, Crafton Hills College (CA); Sandra Scheller, Wayland Baptist University (TX); Sandra Schroeder, Yakima Valley College (WA); Holly Schullo, University of Louisiana, Lafayette; Gloria Scott, Towson University (MD); Laine Scott, La Grange College (GA); Aparna Screenivasan, California State University, Monterey Bay; Michael Sewell, Wayland Baptist University (TX); Jolly Sharp, Cumberland College (KY); Meighan Sharp, Emory and Henry College (VA); Amy Sheldon, SUNY Geneseo (NY); Brandi Shelton, Nashville State Technical Community College (TN); Suzanne Shepard, Broome Community College (NY); Jean Sheridan, University of Southern Maine, Portland; John Silva, LaGuardia Community College (NY); Mary Beth Simmons, Villanova University (PA); Michele Singletary, Nashville State Technical Community College (TN); Beverly Six, Sul Ross State University (TX); Greta Skogseth, Montcalm Community College (MI); Bonnie Smith, Belmont University (TN); Mary Lou Smith, Alexandria Technical University (MN); Sally Smith, Alexandria Technical University (MN); Sean Smith, Ivy Technical Sate College (IN); James Southerland, Brenau College (GA); Sis Spencer, Trinidad State Junior College (CO); Barbara Steele, Towson University (MD); Sharon Steinberg, Tunxis Community College (CT); Lisa Steinman, Reed College (OR); Shari Stenberg, Creighton University (NE); Rebecca Suarez, University of Texas, El Paso; Jo Suzuki, Master's College and Seminary (CA); Kristine Swenson, University of Missouri, Rolla; Peggy Szczesniak, Genessee Community College (NY); Cynthia Taber, Schenectady County Community College (NY); Dean Taciuch, George Mason University (VA); Marguerite Tassi, University of Nebraska, Kearney; Lisa Terasa, Mount Mary College (WI); Matt Theado, Gardner-Webb University (NC); Catherine Thomas, College of Charleston (SC); Cliff Toliver, Missouri Southern State University; Jill Tucker,

San Diego Miramar College (CA); Anita Turpin, Roanoke College (VA); Pat Tyrer, West Texas A&M University; Wanda Umber, Wayland Baptist University (TX); Kim Van Alkamade, Shippensburg University (PA); Thomas Varner, J. Sargeant Reynolds Community College (VA); Angela Vogel, John Tyler Community College (VA); Michelle Von Euw, University of Maryland; Peter Vose, Falmouth High School (ME); Elizabeth Wagoner, Kent State University (OH); Ralph Wahlstrom, SUNY Buffalo (NY); Shelton Waldrep, University of Southern Maine; Teri Waters, Waubonsee Community College (IL); Pamela Watkins, Los Angeles Harbor Community College (CA); Cindy Welch, Carthage College (WI); Vicky Westacott, Alfred University (NY); Jennifer Whetham, Greenriver Community College (WA); Anne Whitney, University of California, Santa Barbara; John Wiltbank, Tidewater Community College (VA); Barbara Winborn, Asbury College (KY); Rosemary Winslow, Catholic University of America (DC); Kelli Wood-Mancha, El Paso Community College (TX); Michael Woodruff, Hargrave Military Academy (VA); Donna Y. Smith, Wayland Baptist University (OK); Ann Yearick, Radford University (VA); Julie Yen, California State University, Sacramento; Jonathan Ying, Cornell University (NY); Joann Yost, Bethel University (MN); Ben Young, Oregon State University; Michael Young, La Roche College (PA); Laura Zam, George Mason University (VA); Robbin Zeff, George Washington University (DC); Trudy Zimmerman, Hutchinson Community College (KS)

Student contributors

We are indebted to the students whose essays appear in this edition — Ned Bishop, Anna Orlov, Emilia Sanchez, Jamal Hammond, and Luisa Mirano — not only for permission to use their work but also for allowing us to adapt it for pedagogical purposes. Our thanks also go to the students who granted permission to use their paragraphs: Rosa Broderick, Connie Hailey, Craig Lee Hetherington, Kathleen Lewis, Laurie McDonough, Kevin Smith, Margaret Smith, Margaret Stack, and David Warren.

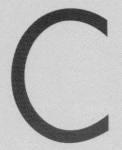

Composing
and Revising

C Composing and Revising

Writing is not a matter of recording already developed thoughts but a process of figuring out what you think. Since it's not possible to think about everything all at once, most experienced writers handle a piece of writing in stages. You will generally move from planning to drafting to revising, but be prepared to return to earlier stages as your ideas develop.

C1

Planning

C1-a Assess the writing situation.

Begin by taking a look at the writing situation in which you find yourself. Consider your subject, the sources of information available to you, your purpose, your audience, and constraints such as length, document design, review sessions, and deadlines or other assignment requirements. It is likely that you will make final decisions about all of these matters later in the writing process — after a first draft, for example. Nevertheless, you can save yourself time by thinking about as many of them as possible in advance. For a quick checklist, see page 5.

ACADEMIC ENGLISH What counts as good writing varies from culture to culture and even among groups within cultures. In some situations, you will need to become familiar with the writing styles — such as direct or indirect, personal or impersonal, plain or embellished—that are valued by the culture or discourse community for which you are writing.

C1-b Experiment with ways to explore your subject.

Instead of just plunging into a first draft, experiment with one or more techniques for exploring your subject — perhaps talking and listening, annotating texts and taking notes, listing, clustering, freewriting, or asking the journalist's questions. Whatever technique you turn to, the goal is the same: to generate a wealth of ideas that will lead you to a question, a problem, or an issue that you want to explore further. At this early stage of the writing process, don't censor yourself. Sometimes an idea that initially seems trivial or far-fetched will turn out to be worthwhile.

Understanding an assignment

Determining the purpose of the assignment

Usually the wording of an assignment will suggest its purpose. You might be expected to do one of the following:

- summarize information from textbooks, lectures, or research
- analyze ideas and concepts
- take a position on a topic and defend it with evidence
- create an original argument by combining ideas from different sources

Understanding how to answer an assignment's questions

Many assignments will ask a *how* or *why* question. Such a question cannot be answered using only facts; you will need to take a position. For example, the question "What are the survival rates for leukemia patients?" can be answered by reporting facts. The question "Why are the survival rates for leukemia patients in one state lower than in a neighboring state?" must be answered with both facts and interpretation.

If a list of prompts appears in the assignment, be careful — instructors rarely expect you to answer all of the questions in order. Look instead for topics, themes, or ideas that will help you ask your own questions.

Recognizing implied questions

When an assignment asks you to *discuss, analyze, agree or disagree,* or *consider* a topic, your instructor will often expect you to answer a *how* or *why* question. For example, "*Discuss* the effects of the No Child Left Behind Act on special education programs" is another way of saying "*How* has the No Child Left Behind Act affected special education programs?" Similarly, the assignment "*Consider* the recent rise of attention deficit hyperactivity disorder diagnoses" is asking you to answer the question "*Why* are diagnoses of attention deficit hyperactivity disorder rising?"

ON THE WEB > dianahacker.com/writersref
Writing exercises > E-ex C1–1

ON THE WEB > dianahacker.com/writersref
Additional resources > Links Library > Composing and revising

Checklist for assessing the writing situation

Subject

- Has a subject (or a range of possible subjects) been given to you, or are you free to choose your own?
- What interests you about your subject? What questions would you like to explore?
- How broadly can you cover the subject? Do you need to narrow it to a more specific topic (because of length restrictions, for instance)?

Sources of information

- Where will your information come from: Reading? Personal experience? Direct observation? Interviews? Questionnaires?
- What sort of documentation is required?

Purpose and audience

- Why are you writing: To inform readers? To persuade them? To entertain them? To call them to action? Some combination of these?
- Who are your readers? How well informed are they about your subject? How will they benefit from reading your work?
- How interested and attentive are your readers? Will they care about your purpose? Will they resist any of your ideas?
- What is your relationship to them: Student to instructor? Employee to supervisor? Citizen to citizen? Expert to novice? Scholar to scholar?

Length and document design

- Do you have any length specifications? If not, what length seems appropriate, given your subject, purpose, and audience?
- Must you use a particular format for your document? If so, do you have guidelines to follow or examples to consult?

Reviewers and deadlines

- Who will be reviewing your draft in progress: Your instructor? A writing center tutor? Your classmates? A friend? Someone in your family?
- What are your deadlines? How much time will you need to allow for the various stages of writing, including proofreading and printing the final draft?

Talking and listening

Since writing is a process of figuring out what you think about a subject, it can be useful to try out your ideas on other people. Conversation can deepen and refine your ideas before you even begin to set them down on paper. By talking and listening to others, you can also discover what they find interesting, what they are curious about, and where they disagree with you. If you are planning to advance an argument, you can try it out on listeners with other points of view.

Many writers begin by brainstorming ideas in a group, debating a point with friends, or chatting with an instructor. Others turn to themselves for company — by talking into a tape recorder. Some writers exchange ideas by sending e-mails or instant messages, by joining an Internet chat group, or by following a mailing list discussion. If you are part of a networked classroom, you may be encouraged to share ideas with others in an electronic workshop. For example, a student who participated in the following chat was able to refine her argument before she started drafting her essay on presidential campaign funding.

CONVERSATION ABOUT A SUBJECT

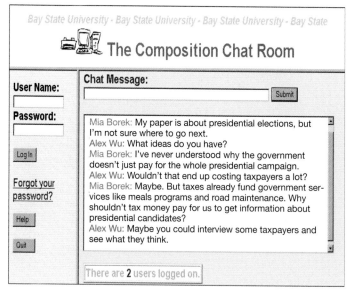

Annotating texts

When you write about reading, one of the best ways to explore ideas is to mark up the work — on the pages themselves if you own the work, on photocopies or sticky notes if you don't. Annotating a text encourages you to look at it more carefully — to underline key concepts, to note possible contradictions in an argument, to raise questions for further investigation. Here, for example, is a paragraph from an essay on medical ethics as one student annotated it:

What break-
throughs?
Do all break-
throughs have
the same
consequences?

Breakthroughs in genetics present us with a promise and a predicament. The promise is that we may soon be able to treat and prevent a host of debilitating diseases. The predicament is that our newfound genetic knowledge may also enable us *Stem cell* to manipulate our own nature — to enhance our *research?* muscles, memories, and moods; to choose the sex, height, and other genetic traits of our children; to make ourselves "better than well." When science moves faster than (moral understanding) as it does *What does he* today, men and women struggle to articulate their *mean by "moral*

Is everyone
really uneasy?
Is something a
breakthrough if
it creates a
predicament?

unease. In liberal societies they reach first for the *understanding"?* language of autonomy, fairness, and individual rights. But this part of our moral vocabulary is ill equipped to address the hardest questions posed *Which ques-* by genetic engineering. The genomic revolution *tions? He* has induced a kind of moral vertigo. *doesn't seem to*
— Michael Sandel, "The Case against Perfection" *be taking sides.*

Listing

Listing ideas is a good way to figure out what you know and what questions you have. You might simply write ideas in the order in which they occur to you — a technique sometimes known as *brainstorming.* Here is a list one student writer jotted down for an essay about funding for college athletics:

Football receives the most funding of any sport.

Funding comes from ticket sales, fundraisers, alumni contributions.

Biggest women's sport is soccer.

Women's soccer team is only ten years old; football team is fifty years old.

Football graduates have had time to earn more money than soccer graduates.

Soccer games don't draw as many fans.

Should funding be equal for all teams?

Do alumni have the right to fund whatever they want?

Feel free to rearrange ideas, to group them under general categories, to delete some, and to add others. In other words, treat the initial list as a source of ideas and a springboard to new ideas, not as an outline.

Clustering

Unlike listing, the technique of clustering highlights relationships among ideas. To cluster ideas, write your topic in the center of a sheet of paper, draw a circle around it, and surround that circle with related ideas connected to it with lines. If some of the satellite ideas lead to more specific clusters, write them down as well. The writer of the following cluster diagram was exploring ideas for an essay on obesity in children.

CLUSTER DIAGRAM

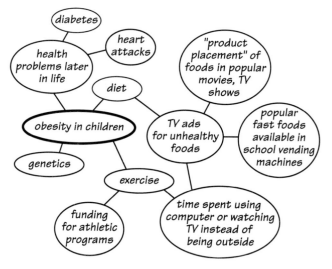

ON THE WEB > dianahacker.com/writersref
Resources for writers and tutors > Tips from writing tutors:
Invention strategies

Freewriting

In its purest form, freewriting is simply nonstop writing. You set aside ten minutes or so and write whatever comes to you, without pausing to think about word choice, spelling, or even meaning. If you get stuck, you can write about being stuck, but you should keep your fingers moving. If nothing much happens, you have lost only ten minutes. It's more likely, though, that something interesting will emerge — an eloquent sentence, an honest expression of feeling, or an idea worth further investigation. To explore ideas on a particular topic, consider using a technique called *focused freewriting*. Again, you write quickly and freely, but this time you focus on a subject and pay attention to the connections among your ideas.

Asking the journalist's questions

By asking relevant questions, you can generate many ideas — and you can make sure that you have adequately surveyed your subject. When gathering material for a story, journalists routinely ask themselves Who? What? When? Where? Why? and How? In addition to helping journalists get started, these questions ensure that they will not overlook an important fact: the date of a prospective summit meeting, for example, or the exact location of a burglary.

Whenever you are writing about events, whether current or historical, asking the journalist's questions is one way to get started. One student, whose subject was the negative reaction in 1915 to D. W. Griffith's silent film *The Birth of a Nation*, began exploring her topic with this set of questions:

Who objected to the film?

What were the objections?

When were the protests first voiced?

Where were protests most strongly expressed?

Why did protesters object to the film?

How did protesters make their views known?

In the academic world, scholars often generate ideas with questions related to a specific discipline: one set of questions for analyzing short stories, another for evaluating experiments in social psychology, still another for reporting field experiences in anthropology. If you are writing in a particular discipline, try to discover the questions that its scholars typically explore (see A4).

C1-c Formulate a tentative thesis.

As you explore your subject and identify questions you would like to investigate, you will begin to see possible ways to focus your material. At this point, try to settle on a tentative central idea. The more complex your topic, the more your focus will change as your drafts evolve.

For many types of writing, you will be able to assert your central idea in a sentence or two. Such a statement, which ordinarily appears in the opening paragraph of your finished essay, is called a *thesis* (see also C2-a). A thesis is often the answer to a question, the resolution of a problem, or a statement that takes a position on a debatable topic. A successful thesis — like the following, all taken from articles in *Smithsonian* magazine — points both the writer and the reader in a definite direction.

> Much maligned and the subject of unwarranted fears, most bats are harmless and highly beneficial.

> The American Revolution was the central event in Washington's life, the crucible for his development as a mature man, a prominent statesman, and a national hero.

> Raging in mines from Pennsylvania to China, coal fires threaten towns, poison air and water, and add to global warming.

The thesis sentence usually contains a key word or controlling idea that limits its focus. The first two example sentences, for instance, use key words to prepare for essays that focus on the *beneficial* aspects of bats and the role of the American Revolution in the *development* of George Washington. The third example uses a controlling idea: the *effects* of coal fires.

It's a good idea to formulate a tentative thesis early in the writing process, perhaps by jotting it on scratch paper, by putting it at the head of a rough outline, or by drafting an introductory paragraph that includes it. This tentative thesis will help you shape your thoughts. Don't worry about the exact wording because your main point may change as you refine your ideas. Here, for example, is one student's early effort:

> In *Rebel without a Cause*, the protagonist, Jim Stark, is often seen literally on the edge of physical danger — walking too close to the swimming pool, leaning over an observation deck, and driving his car toward a cliff.

The thesis that appeared in the student's final draft not only was more polished but also reflected the evolution of the student's ideas.

Testing a tentative thesis

- Is the thesis too obvious? If you cannot come up with interpretations that oppose your own, consider revising your thesis.
- Can you support your thesis with the evidence available?
- Does the thesis require an essay's worth of development? Or will you run out of points too quickly?
- Can you explain why readers will want to read an essay with this thesis?

The scenes in which Jim Stark is seen on the edge of physical danger — walking too close to the swimming pool, leaning over an observation deck, driving his car toward a cliff — suggest that he is becoming more and more agitated by the constraints of family and society.

For a more detailed discussion of thesis, see C2-a.

C1-d Sketch a plan.

Once you have generated some ideas and formulated a tentative thesis, you might want to sketch an informal outline to see how you will support your thesis and to begin to structure your ideas. Informal outlines can take many forms. Perhaps the most common is simply the thesis followed by a list of major ideas.

Thesis: Television advertising should be regulated to help prevent childhood obesity.

- Children watch more television than ever.
- Snacks marketed to children are often unhealthy and fattening.
- Childhood obesity can cause diabetes and other health problems.
- Solving these health problems costs taxpayers billions of dollars.
- Therefore, these ads are actually costing the public money.
- But if advertising is free speech, do we have the right to regulate it?
- We regulate liquor and cigarette ads on television, so why not advertising aimed at children?

If you began by jotting down a list of ideas or drawing a clustering diagram, you may be able to turn that list or diagram into a rough outline by crossing out some ideas, adding others, and putting the ideas in a logical order.

When to use a formal outline

Early in the writing process, rough outlines have certain advantages over their more formal counterparts: They can be produced more quickly, they are more obviously tentative, and they can be revised more easily should the need arise. However, a formal outline may be useful later in the writing process, after you have written a rough draft, especially if your subject matter is complex.

The following formal outline brought order to the research paper that appears in MLA-5b, on Internet surveillance in the workplace. Notice that the student's thesis is an important part of the outline. Everything else in the outline supports it, directly or indirectly.

> Thesis: Although companies often have legitimate concerns that lead them to monitor employees' Internet usage — from expensive security breaches to reduced productivity — the benefits of electronic surveillance are outweighed by its costs to employees' privacy and autonomy.
>
> I. Although employers have always monitored employees, electronic surveillance is more efficient.
>   A. Employers can gather data in large quantities.
>   B. Electronic surveillance can be continuous.
>   C. Electronic surveillance can be conducted secretly, with keystroke logging programs.
>
> II. Some experts argue that employers have legitimate reasons to monitor employees' Internet usage.
>   A. Unmonitored employees could accidentally breach security.
>   B. Companies are legally accountable for online actions of employees.
>
> III. Despite valid concerns, employers should value employee morale and autonomy and avoid creating an atmosphere of distrust.
>   A. Setting the boundaries for employee autonomy is difficult in the wired workplace.
>   1. Using the Internet is the most popular way of wasting time at work.
>   2. Employers can't tell easily if employees are working or surfing the Web.
>   B. Surveillance can create resentment among employees.
>   1. Web surfing can relieve stress, and restricting it can generate tension between managers and workers.
>   2. Enforcing Internet usage can seem arbitrary.

IV. Surveillance may not increase employee productivity, and trust may benefit it.

    A. It shouldn't matter to the company how many hours salaried employees work as long as they get the job done.

    B. Casual Internet use can actually benefit companies.

       1. The Internet may spark business ideas.

       2. The Internet may suggest ideas about how to operate more efficiently.

V. Employees' rights to privacy are not well defined by the law.

    A. Few federal guidelines exist on electronic surveillance.

    B. Employers and employees are negotiating the boundaries without legal guidance.

    C. As technological capabilities increase, there will be an increased need to define boundaries.

Guidelines for constructing an outline

1. Put the thesis at the top.

2. Make items at the same level of generality as parallel as possible (see S1).

3. Use sentences unless phrases are clear.

4. Use the conventional system of numbers and letters for the levels of generality.

    I.

      A.

      B.

        1.

        2.

          a.

          b.

    II.

5. Always use at least two subdivisions for a category, since nothing can be divided into fewer than two parts.

6. Limit the number of major sections in the outline; if the list of roman numerals begins to look like a laundry list, find some way of clustering the items into a few major categories with more subcategories.

7. Be flexible; in other words, be prepared to change your outline as your drafts evolve.

C2

Drafting

As you rough out an initial draft, focus your attention on ideas and organization. You can think about sentence structure and word choice later. Writing tends to flow better when it is drafted relatively quickly, without many stops and starts. Keep your prewriting materials — lists, outlines, freewriting, and so on — close at hand. In addition to helping you get started, such notes and blueprints will encourage you to keep moving.

For most kinds of writing, an introduction announces the main point, the body paragraphs develop it, and the conclusion drives it home. You can begin drafting, however, at any point. If you find it difficult to introduce a paper that you have not yet written, try drafting the body first and saving the introduction for later.

ON THE WEB > dianahacker.com/writersref
Resources for writers and tutors > Tips from writing tutors:
Writing introductions and conclusions

C2-a For most types of writing, draft an introduction that includes a thesis.

Your introduction will usually be a paragraph of 50 to 150 words (in a longer paper, it may be more than one paragraph). Perhaps the most common strategy is to open the paragraph with a few sentences that engage the reader, establish your purpose for writing, and conclude with your main point. The sentence stating the main point is called a *thesis*. (See also C1-c.) In the following examples, the thesis has been italicized.

> Credit card companies love to extend credit to college students, especially those just out of high school. Ads for credit cards line campus bulletin boards, flash across commercial Web sites for students, and get stuffed into shopping bags at college bookstores. Why do the companies market their product so vigorously to a population that lacks a substantial credit history and often has no steady source of income? The answer is that significant profits can be earned through high interest rates and assorted penalties and fees. *By granting college students liberal lending arrangements, credit card companies often hook them on a cycle of spending that can ultimately lead to financial ruin.*   — Matt Watson, student

As the United States industrialized in the nineteenth century, using desperate immigrant labor, social concerns took a backseat to the task of building a prosperous nation. The government did not regulate industries and did not provide an effective safety net for the poor or for those who became sick or injured on the job. Luckily, immigrants and the poor did have a few advocates. Settlement houses such as Hull-House in Chicago provided information, services, and a place for reform-minded individuals to gather and work to improve the conditions of the urban poor. Alice Hamilton was one of these reformers. *Hamilton's efforts helped to improve the lives of immigrants and drew attention and respect to the problems and people that until then had been virtually ignored.*

— Laurie McDonough, student

Ideally, the sentences leading to the thesis should hook the reader, perhaps with one of the following:

a startling statistic, an unusual fact, or a vivid example

a paradoxical statement

a quotation or a bit of dialogue

a question

an analogy

an anecdote

Whether you are writing for a scholarly audience, a professional audience, or a general audience, you cannot assume your readers' interest in the topic. The hook should spark curiosity and offer readers a reason to continue reading.

Although the thesis frequently appears at the end of the introduction, it can also appear at the beginning. Much work-related writing, in which a straightforward approach is most effective, commonly begins with the thesis.

Flextime scheduling, which has proved its effectiveness at the Library of Congress, should be introduced on a trial basis at the main branch of the Montgomery County Public Library. By offering flexible work hours, the library can boost employee morale, cut down on absenteeism, and expand its hours of operation.

— David Warren, student

For some types of writing, it may be difficult or impossible to express the central idea in a thesis sentence; or it may be unwise or unnecessary to put a thesis sentence in the essay itself. A personal narrative, for example, may have a focus too subtle to be distilled in a single sentence, and such a sentence might ruin the story. Strictly informative writing, like that found in many business memos, may be difficult to summarize in a thesis. In such instances, do not try to force the central idea into a thesis sentence. Instead, think in terms of an overriding purpose, which may or may not be stated directly.

> ACADEMIC ENGLISH If you come from a culture that prefers an indirect approach in writing, you may feel that asserting a thesis early in an essay sounds unrefined or even rude. In the United States, however, readers appreciate a direct approach; when you state your point as directly as possible, you show that you value your readers' time.

Characteristics of an effective thesis

An effective thesis sentence is a central idea that requires supporting evidence; it is of adequate scope for an essay of the assigned length; and it is sharply focused.

A thesis must require proof or further development through facts and details; it cannot itself be a fact or a description.

TOO FACTUAL   The polygraph was developed by Dr. John A. Larson in 1921.

REVISED   Because the polygraph has not been proved reliable, even under controlled conditions, its use by employers should be banned.

A thesis should be of sufficient scope for your assignment, not too broad and not too narrow. Unless you are writing a book or a very long research paper, the following thesis is too broad.

TOO BROAD   Mapping the human genome has many implications for health and science.

REVISED   Although scientists can now detect genetic predisposition to specific diseases, not everyone should be tested for these diseases.

A thesis should be sharply focused, not too vague. Avoid fuzzy, hard-to-define words such as *interesting, good,* or *disgusting.*

TOO VAGUE   The way the TV show *ER* portrays doctors and nurses is interesting.

REVISED   In dramatizing the experiences of doctors and nurses as they treat patients, navigate medical bureaucracy, and negotiate bioethical dilemmas, the TV show *ER* portrays health care professionals as unfailingly caring and noble.

In the process of making a too-vague thesis more precise, you may find yourself outlining the major sections of your paper, as in the preceding example. This technique, known as *blueprinting*, helps readers know exactly what to expect as they read on. It also helps you, the writer, control the shape of your essay.

ON THE WEB > dianahacker.com/writersref
Writing exercises > E-ex C2–1 and C2–2

C2-b Draft the body.

The body of an essay develops support for a thesis, so it's important to have at least a tentative thesis before you start writing. What does your thesis promise readers? Try to keep your response to that question in mind as you draft the body.

If you have sketched a preliminary plan, try to block out your paragraphs accordingly. If you do not have a plan, you would be wise to pause a moment and sketch one (see C1-d). Keep in mind that often you might not know what you want to say until you have written a draft. It is possible to begin without a plan — assuming you are prepared to treat your first attempt as a "discovery draft" that will almost certainly be tossed or rewritten once you discover what you really want to say.

For more advice about paragraphs and paragraphing, see C4.

C2-c Draft a conclusion.

A conclusion should remind readers of the essay's main idea without dully repeating it. Often the concluding paragraph can be relatively short. By the end of the essay, readers should already understand your main point; your conclusion simply drives it home and, perhaps, leaves readers with something larger to consider.

In addition to echoing your main idea, a conclusion might briefly summarize the essay's key points, propose a course of action, discuss the topic's wider significance, offer advice, or pose a question for future study. To conclude an essay analyzing the shifting roles of women in the military services, one student discusses her topic's implications for society as a whole:

> As the military continues to train women in jobs formerly reserved for men, our understanding of women's roles in society will no doubt continue to change. When news reports of women

training for and taking part in combat operations become commonplace, reports of women becoming CEOs, police chiefs, and even president of the United States will cease to surprise us. Or perhaps we have already reached this point.   — Rosa Broderick, student

To make the conclusion memorable, you might include a detail, an example, or an image from the introduction to bring readers full circle; a quotation or a bit of dialogue; an anecdote; or a humorous or ironic comment.

Whatever concluding strategy you choose, keep in mind that an effective conclusion is decisive and unapologetic. Avoid introducing wholly new ideas at the end of an essay. Finally, because the conclusion is so closely tied to the rest of the essay in both content and tone, be prepared to rework it (or even replace it) when you revise.

C3

Revising

Revising is rarely a one-step process. Global matters — focus, purpose, organization, content, and overall strategy — generally receive attention first. Improvements in sentence structure, word choice, grammar, punctuation, and mechanics come later.

C3-a Make global revisions.

By the time you've written a draft, your ideas will probably have gone in directions you couldn't have predicted ahead of time. As a result, global revisions can be quite dramatic. It's possible, for example, that your thesis will evolve as you figure out how your ideas fit together. You might drop whole paragraphs and add others or condense material once stretched over two or three paragraphs. You might rearrange entire sections. You will save time if you handle global revisions before turning to sentence-level issues: There is little sense in revising sentences that may not appear in your final draft.

Many of us resist global revisions because we find it difficult to view our work from our audience's perspective. To distance yourself from a draft, put it aside for a while, preferably overnight or longer. When you return to it, try to play the role of your audience as you

EXAMPLE OF GLOBAL REVISIONS

Big Box Stores Aren't So Bad

In her essay Big Box Stores Are Bad for Main Street, Betsy Taylor shifts

the focus away from the economic effects of these stores to the effects

these stores have on the "soul" of America. She claims that stores like Home

Depot and Target are bad for America, they draw people out of downtown

shopping districts and cause them to focus exclusively on consumption. She

believes that small businesses are good for America because they provide

personal attention, foster community interaction, and make each city

different from the other ones. But Taylor's argument is not strong because it

is based on nostalgic images rather than true assumptions about the roles

that businesses play in consumers lives and communities. Taylor reveals that

she has a nostalgic view of American society and does not understand

economic realities. ~~She focuses~~ on idealized shoppers and shopkeepers

interacting on the quaint Main Streets of America rather than the eco-

nomic realities of the situation. As a result, she incorrectly assumes that

simply getting rid of big box stores would have a positive effect on us.

For example, in her first paragraph she refers to a big box store as a

"25-acre slab of concrete with a 100,000 square foot box of stuff" that lands

on a town, evoking images of something strong and powerful conquering

something small and weak. But she oversimplifies a complex issue.

*She ignores the more complex and economically driven relation-
ship between large chain stores and the communities in which
they exist.*

read. If possible, enlist the help of reviewers — persons willing to
read your draft, focusing on the larger issues, not on the fine points.
The checklist for global revision on page 21 may help them get
started.

EXAMPLE OF SENTENCE-LEVEL REVISIONS

Rethinking Big-Box Stores
~~Big Box Stores Aren't So Bad~~

In her essay *"*Big Box Stores Are Bad for Main Street*,"* Betsy Taylor ~~shifts~~
focuses not on *large chain* *but on*
~~the focus away from~~ the economic effects of ~~these~~ stores ~~to~~ the effects these

argues
stores have on the "soul" of America. She ~~claims~~ that stores like Home Depot*,*
and Wal-Mart *because*
~~and~~ Target*,* are bad for America*/* ~~they~~ draw people out of downtown shopping
In contrast, she
districts and cause them to focus exclusively on consumption. ~~She~~ believes

that small businesses are good for America because they provide personal

unique.
attention, foster community interaction, and make each city ~~different from~~
ultimately unconvincing
~~the other ones.~~ But Taylor's argument is ~~not strong~~ because it is based on

nostalgia *images of a*
~~nostalgic images~~--on idealized ~~shoppers and shopkeepers interacting on the~~
on
quaint Main Street*s* ~~of America~~--rather than ~~true assumptions about~~ the roles
, *By ignoring*
that businesses play in consumers lives and communities. ~~She ignores~~ the

more complex*,* ~~and~~ economically driven relationship between large chain stores
their *Taylor*
and ~~the~~ communities*,* ~~in which they exist. As a result, she~~ incorrectly assumes
- *America's communities.*
that simply getting rid of big box stores would have a positive effect on ~~us.~~
Taylor's colorful use of language
~~Taylor~~ reveals that she has a nostalgic view of American society and does
In *Taylor*
not understand economic realities. ~~For example, in~~ her first paragraph*,* ~~she~~
-
refers to a big box store as a "25-acre slab of concrete with a 100,000 square
a monolithic
foot box of stuff*"* that *"*lands on a town*,"* evoking images of ~~something strong~~
monster crushing the American way of life (1011).
~~and powerful conquering something small and weak.~~ But she oversimplifies

a complex issue.

TIP: When working on a computer, you might want to print out a hard copy and read the draft as a whole rather than screen by screen. Once you have decided what global revisions may be needed, the computer is an excellent tool for combining or rearranging paragraphs. With little risk, you can explore the possibilities. When a revision misfires, it is easy to return to your original draft.

ON THE WEB > dianahacker.com/writersref
   Writing exercises > E-ex C3–1

Checklist for global revision

Purpose and audience

- Does the draft accomplish its purpose — to inform readers, to persuade them, to entertain them, to call them to action?
- Is the draft appropriate for its audience? Does it account for the audience's knowledge of the subject, level of interest in the subject, and possible attitudes toward the subject?

Focus

- Is the thesis clear? Is it placed prominently? If there is no thesis, is there a good reason for omitting one?
- Do the introduction and conclusion focus clearly on the central idea?
- Are any ideas obviously off the point?

Organization and paragraphing

- Are there enough organizational cues for readers (such as topic sentences or headings)?
- Are ideas presented in a logical order?
- Are any paragraphs too long or too short for easy reading?

Content

- Is the supporting material relevant and persuasive?
- Which ideas need further development?
- Are the parts proportioned sensibly? Do major ideas receive enough attention?
- Where might material be deleted?

Point of view

- Is the draft free of distracting shifts in point of view (from *I* to *you*, for example, or from *it* to *they*)?
- Is the dominant point of view — first person (*I* or *we*), second person (*you*), or third person (*he, she, it, one,* or *they*) — appropriate for your purpose and audience? (See S4-a.)

ON THE WEB > dianahacker.com/writersref
Writing exercises > E-ex C3–2

ON THE WEB > dianahacker.com/writersref
Resources for writers and tutors > Tips from writing tutors:
Revising and editing

C3-b Revise and edit sentences.

Much of the rest of this book offers advice on revising sentences for style and clarity and on editing them for grammar, punctuation, and mechanics. Some writers handle sentence-level revisions directly at the computer, experimenting on-screen with a variety of improvements. Other writers prefer to print out a hard copy of the draft, mark it up, and then return to the computer. Here, for example, is a draft paragraph edited for a variety of sentence-level problems.

Although some cities have found creative ways to improve access to public transportation for physically handicapped passengers, ~~and to fund other programs, there have been problems in~~ our city has struggled with ~~due to the need to address~~ budget constraints and competing ~~needs~~ priorities. ~~This~~ The budget crunch has led citizens to question how funds are distributed. ~~?~~ For example, last year ~~when~~ city officials voted to use available funds to support ~~had to choose between allocating funds for accessible transportation or allocating funds to~~ after-school programs rather than transportation upgrades. ~~, they voted for the after-school programs.~~ It is not clear to some citizens why ~~these~~ after-school programs are more important.

The original paragraph was flawed by wordiness, a problem that can be addressed through any number of revisions. This revision would also be acceptable:

> Some cities have funded improved access to public transportation for physically handicapped passengers. Because of budget constraints, our city chose to fund after-school programs rather than transportation programs. As a result, citizens have begun to question how funds are distributed and why certain programs are more important than others.

Some of the paragraph's improvements are not open to debate and must be fixed in any revision. The hyphen in *after-school programs* is necessary; a noun must be substituted for the pronoun *these* in the last sentence; and the question mark in the second sentence must be changed to a period.

> ✓ GRAMMAR CHECKERS can help with some but by no means all of the sentence-level problems in a typical draft. Many problems — such as faulty parallelism and misplaced modifiers — require an understanding of grammatical structure that computer programs lack. Such problems often slip right past the grammar checker. Even when the grammar checker makes a suggestion for revision, it is your responsibility as the writer to decide whether the suggestion is more effective than your original.

C3-c Proofread the final manuscript.

After revising and editing, you are ready to prepare the final manuscript. (See C5.) Make sure to allow yourself enough time for proofreading — the final and most important step in manuscript preparation.

Proofreading is a special kind of reading: a slow and methodical search for misspellings, typographical mistakes, and omitted words or word endings. Such errors can be difficult to spot in your own work because you may read what you intended to write, not what is actually on the page. To fight this tendency, try proofreading out loud, articulating each word as it is actually written. You might also try proofreading your sentences in reverse order, a strategy that takes your attention away from the meanings you intended and forces you to focus on one word at a time.

Although proofreading may be dull, it is crucial. Errors strewn throughout an essay are distracting and annoying. A reader may think, If the writer doesn't care about this piece of writing, why should I? A carefully proofread essay, however, sends the message that you value your writing and respect your readers.

> ✓ SPELL CHECKERS are more reliable than grammar checkers, but they too must be used with caution. Many typographical errors (such as *quiet* for *quite*) and misused words (such as *effect* for *affect*) slip past the spell checker because the checker flags only words not found in its dictionary.

ON THE WEB > dianahacker.com/writersref
Model papers > MLA paper-in-progress: Watson

C4

Writing paragraphs

Except for special-purpose paragraphs, such as introductions and conclusions (see C2-a and C2-c), paragraphs are clusters of information supporting an essay's main point (or advancing a story's action). Aim for paragraphs that are clearly focused, well developed, organized, coherent, and neither too long nor too short for easy reading.

C4-a Focus on a main point.

A paragraph should be unified around a main point. The point should be clear to readers, and all sentences in the paragraph should relate to it.

Stating the main point in a topic sentence

As a rule, you should state the main point of a paragraph in a topic sentence — a one-sentence summary that tells readers what to expect as they read on. Usually the topic sentence comes first in the paragraph.

> *All living creatures manage some form of communication.* The dance patterns of bees in their hive help to point the way to distant flower fields or announce successful foraging. Male stickleback fish regularly swim upside-down to indicate outrage in a courtship contest. Male deer and lemurs mark territorial ownership by rubbing their own body secretions on boundary stones or trees. Everyone has seen a frightened dog put his tail between his legs and run in panic. We, too, use gestures, expressions, postures, and movement to give our words point. [Italics added.]
> — Olivia Vlahos, *Human Beginnings*

Sometimes the topic sentence is introduced by a transitional sentence linking the paragraph to earlier material, and occasionally it is withheld until the end of the paragraph. And at times a topic sentence is not needed: if a paragraph continues developing an idea clearly introduced in an earlier paragraph, if the details of the paragraph unmistakably suggest its main point, or if the paragraph appears in a narrative of events where generalizations might interrupt the flow of the story.

Sticking to the point

Sentences that do not support the topic sentence destroy the unity of a paragraph. If the paragraph is otherwise well focused, such offending sentences can simply be deleted or perhaps moved elsewhere. In the following paragraph describing the inadequate facilities in a high school, the information about the chemistry instructor (in italics) is clearly off the point.

> As the result of tax cuts, the educational facilities of Lincoln High School have reached an all-time low. Some of the books date back to 1990 and have long since shed their covers. The few computers in working order must share one printer. The lack of lab equipment makes it necessary for four or five students to work at one table, with most watching rather than performing experiments. *Also, the chemistry instructor left to have a baby at the beginning of the semester, and most of the students don't like the substitute.* As for the furniture, many of the upright chairs have become recliners, and the desk legs are so unbalanced that they play seesaw on the floor. [Italics added.]

Sometimes the solution for a disunified paragraph is not as simple as deleting or moving material. Writers often wander into uncharted territory because they cannot think of enough evidence to support a topic sentence. Feeling that it is too soon to break into a new paragraph, they move on to new ideas for which they have not prepared the reader. When this happens, the writer is faced with a choice: Either find more evidence to support the topic sentence or adjust the topic sentence to mesh with the evidence that is available.

ON THE WEB > dianahacker.com/writersref
Writing exercises > E-ex C4–1

C4-b Develop the main point.

Though an occasional short paragraph is fine, particularly if it functions as a transition or emphasizes a point, a series of brief paragraphs suggests inadequate development. How much development is enough? That varies, depending on the writer's purpose and audience.

For example, when she wrote a paragraph attempting to convince readers that it is impossible to lose fat quickly, health columnist Jane Brody knew that she would have to present a great deal of evidence because many dieters want to believe the opposite. She did *not* write:

> When you think about it, it's impossible to lose — as many diets suggest — 10 pounds of *fat* in ten days, even on a total fast. Even a moderately active person cannot lose so much weight so fast. A less active person hasn't a prayer.

This three-sentence paragraph is too skimpy to be convincing. But the paragraph that Brody in fact wrote contains enough evidence to convince even skeptical readers.

> When you think about it, it's impossible to lose — as many . . . diets suggest — 10 pounds of *fat* in ten days, even on a total fast. A pound of body fat represents 3,500 calories. To lose 1 pound of fat, you must expend 3,500 more calories than you consume. Let's say you weigh 170 pounds and, as a moderately active person, you burn 2,500 calories a day. If your diet contains only 1,500 calories, you'd have an energy deficit of 1,000 calories a day. In a week's time that would add up to a 7,000-calorie deficit, or 2 pounds of real fat. In ten days, the accumulated deficit would represent nearly 3 pounds of lost body fat. Even if you ate nothing at all for ten days and maintained your usual level of activity, your caloric deficit would add up to 25,000 calories. . . . At 3,500 calories per pound of fat, that's still only 7 pounds of lost fat.
>
> — Jane Brody, *Jane Brody's Nutrition Book*

C4-c Choose a suitable pattern of organization.

Although paragraphs may be patterned in any number of ways, certain patterns of organization occur frequently, either alone or in combination: examples and illustrations, narration, description, process, comparison and contrast, analogy, cause and effect, classification and division, and definition. There is nothing particularly magical about these patterns (sometimes called *methods of development*). They simply reflect some of the ways in which we think.

Examples and illustrations

Examples, perhaps the most common pattern of organization, are appropriate whenever the reader might be tempted to ask, "For example?"

Normally my parents abided scrupulously by "The Budget," but several times a year Dad would dip into his battered black strongbox and splurge on some irrational, totally satisfying luxury. Once he bought over a hundred comic books at a flea market, doled out to us thereafter at the tantalizing rate of two a week. He always got a whole flat of pansies, Mom's favorite flower, for us to give her on Mother's Day. One day a boy stopped at our house selling fifty-cent raffle tickets on a sailboat and Dad bought every ticket the boy had left — three books' worth.

— Connie Hailey, student

Illustrations are extended examples, frequently presented in story form.

Part of [Harriet Tubman's] strategy of conducting was, as in all battle-field operations, the knowledge of how and when to retreat. Numerous allusions have been made to her moves when she suspected that she was in danger. When she feared the party was closely pursued, she would take it for a time on a train southward bound. No one seeing Negroes going in this direction would for an instant suppose them to be fugitives. Once on her return she was at a railroad station. She saw some men reading a poster and she heard one of them reading it aloud. It was a description of her, offering a reward for her capture. She took a southbound train to avert suspicion. At another time when Harriet heard men talking about her, she pretended to read a book which she carried. One man remarked, "This can't be the woman. The one we want can't read or write." Harriet devoutly hoped the book was right side up.

— Earl Conrad, *Harriet Tubman*

Narration

A paragraph of narration tells a story or part of a story. The following paragraph recounts one of the author's experiences in the African wild.

One evening when I was wading in the shallows of the lake to pass a rocky outcrop, I suddenly stopped dead as I saw the sinuous black body of a snake in the water. It was all of six feet long, and from the slight hood and the dark stripes at the back of the neck I knew it to be a Storm's water cobra — a deadly reptile for the bite of which there was, at that time, no serum. As I stared at it an incoming wave gently deposited part of its body on one of my feet. I remained motionless, not even breathing, until the wave rolled back into the lake, drawing the snake with it. Then I leaped out of the water as fast as I could, my heart hammering.

— Jane Goodall, *In the Shadow of Man*

Description

A descriptive paragraph sketches a portrait of a person, place, or thing by using concrete and specific details that appeal to one or more senses — sight, sound, smell, taste, and touch. Consider, for example, the following description of the grasshopper invasions that devastated the midwestern landscape in the late 1860s.

> They came like dive bombers out of the west. They came by the millions with the rustle of their wings roaring overhead. They came in waves, like the rolls of the sea, descending with a terrifying speed, breaking now and again like a mighty surf. They came with the force of a williwaw and they formed a huge, ominous, dark brown cloud that eclipsed the sun. They dipped and touched earth, hitting objects and people like hailstones. But they were not hail. These were *live* demons. They popped, snapped, crackled, and roared. They were dark brown, an inch or longer in length, plump in the middle and tapered at the ends. They had transparent wings, slender legs, and two black eyes that flashed with a fierce intelligence.   — Eugene Boe, "Pioneers to Eternity"

Process

A process paragraph is structured in chronological order. A writer may choose this pattern either to describe how something is made or done or to explain to readers, step by step, how to do something. The following paragraph explains how to perform a "roll cast," a popular fly-fishing technique.

> Begin by taking up a suitable stance, with one foot slightly in front of the other and the rod pointing down the line. Then begin a smooth, steady draw, raising your rod hand to just above shoulder height and lifting the rod to the 10:30 or 11:00 position. This steady draw allows a loop of line to form between the rod top and the water. While the line is still moving, raise the rod slightly, then punch it rapidly forward and down. The rod is now flexed and under maximum compression, and the line follows its path, bellying out slightly behind you and coming off the water close to your feet. As you power the rod down through the 3:00 position, the belly of line will roll forward. Follow through smoothly so that the line unfolds and straightens above the water.
> — *The Dorling Kindersley Encyclopedia of Fishing*

Comparison and contrast

To compare subjects is to draw attention to their similarities, although the word *compare* also has a broader meaning that includes a consideration of differences. To contrast is to focus only on differences.

Whether a paragraph stresses similarities or differences, it may be patterned in one of two ways. The two subjects may be presented one at a time, as in the following paragraph of contrast.

> So Grant and Lee were in complete contrast, representing two diametrically opposed elements in American life. Grant was the modern man emerging; beyond him, ready to come on the stage, was the great age of steel and machinery, of crowded cities and a restless, burgeoning vitality. Lee might have ridden down from the old age of chivalry, lance in hand, silken banner fluttering over his head. Each man was the perfect champion of his cause, drawing both his strengths and his weaknesses from the people he led.
>
> — Bruce Catton, "Grant and Lee: A Study in Contrasts"

Or a paragraph may proceed point by point, treating two subjects together, one aspect at a time. The following paragraph uses the point-by-point method to contrast the writer's experiences in an American high school and an Irish convent.

> Strangely enough, instead of being academically inferior to my American high school, the Irish convent was superior. In my class at home, *Love Story* was considered pretty heavy reading, so imagine my surprise at finding Irish students who could recite passages from *War and Peace*. In high school we complained about having to study *Romeo and Juliet* in one semester, whereas in Ireland we simultaneously studied *Macbeth* and Dickens's *Hard Times*, in addition to writing a composition a day in English class. In high school, I didn't even begin algebra until the ninth grade, while at the convent seventh graders (or their Irish equivalent) were doing calculus and trigonometry.
>
> — Margaret Stack, student

Analogy

Analogies draw comparisons between items that appear to have little in common. In the following paragraph, physician Lewis Thomas draws an analogy between the behavior of ants and that of humans.

> Ants are so much like human beings as to be an embarrassment. They farm fungi, raise aphids as livestock, launch armies into wars, use chemical sprays to alarm and confuse enemies, capture slaves. The families of weaver ants engage in child labor, holding their larvae like shuttles to spin out the thread that sews the leaves together for their fungus gardens. They exchange information ceaselessly. They do everything but watch television.
>
> — Lewis Thomas, "On Societies as Organisms"

Cause and effect

A paragraph may move from cause to effects or from an effect to its causes. The topic sentence in the following paragraph mentions an effect; the rest of the paragraph lists several causes.

> The fantastic water clarity of the Mount Gambier sinkholes results from several factors. The holes are fed from aquifers holding rainwater that fell decades — even centuries — ago, and that has been filtered through miles of limestone. The high level of calcium that limestone adds causes the silty detritus from dead plants and animals to cling together and settle quickly to the bottom. Abundant bottom vegetation in the shallow sinkholes also helps bind the silt. And the rapid turnover of water prohibits stagnation.
>
> — Hillary Hauser, "Exploring a Sunken Realm in Australia"

Classification and division

Classification is the grouping of items into categories according to some consistent principle. The following paragraph classifies species of electric fish.

> Scientists sort electric fishes into three categories. The first comprises the strongly electric species like the marine electric rays or the freshwater African electric catfish and South American electric eel. Known since the dawn of history, these deliver a punch strong enough to stun a human. In recent years, biologists have focused on a second category: weakly electric fish in the South American and African rivers that use tiny voltages for communication and navigation. The third group contains sharks, nonelectric rays and catfish, which do not emit a field but possess sensors that enable them to detect the minute amounts of electricity that leak out of other organisms.
>
> — Anne and Jack Rudloe, "Electric Warfare: The Fish That Kill with Thunderbolts"

Division takes one item and divides it into parts. As with classification, division should be made according to some consistent principle. The following paragraph describes the components that make up a baseball.

> Like the game itself, a baseball is composed of many layers. One of the delicious joys of childhood is to take apart a baseball and examine the wonders within. You begin by removing the red cotton thread and peeling off the leather cover — which comes from the hide of a Holstein cow and has been tanned, cut, printed,

and punched with holes. Beneath the cover is a thin layer of cotton string, followed by several hundred yards of woolen yarn, which makes up the bulk of the ball. Finally, in the middle is a rubber ball, or "pill," which is a little smaller than a golf ball. Slice into the rubber and you'll find the ball's heart — a cork core. The cork is from Portugal, the rubber from southeast Asia, the covers are American, and the balls are assembled in Costa Rica.

— Dan Gutman, *The Way Baseball Works*

Definition

A definition puts a word or concept into a general class and then provides enough details to distinguish it from other members in the same class. In the following paragraph, the writer defines *envy* as a special kind of desire.

Envy is so integral and so painful a part of what animates behavior in market societies that many people have forgotten the full meaning of the word, simplifying it into one of the synonyms of desire. It is that, which may be why it flourishes in market societies: democracies of desire, they might be called, with money for ballots, stuffing permitted. But envy is more or less than desire. It begins with an almost frantic sense of emptiness inside oneself, as if the pump of one's heart were sucking on air. One has to be blind to perceive the emptiness, of course, but that's just what envy is, a selective blindness. *Invidia*, Latin for envy, translates as "non-sight," and Dante has the envious plodding along under cloaks of lead, their eyes sewn shut with leaden wire. What they are blind to is what they have, God-given and humanly nurtured, in themselves.

— Nelson W. Aldrich Jr., *Old Money*

C4-d   Make paragraphs coherent.

When sentences and paragraphs flow from one to another without discernible bumps, gaps, or shifts, they are said to be coherent. Coherence can be improved by strengthing the various ties between old information and new. A number of techniques for strengthening those ties are detailed in this section.

Linking ideas clearly

Readers expect to learn a paragraph's main point in a topic sentence early in the paragraph. Then, as they move into the body of the paragraph, they expect to encounter specific facts, details, or examples that support the topic sentence — either directly or indirectly. Consider the following paragraph, in which all of the sentences following the topic sentence directly support it.

> A passenger list of the early years [of the Orient Express] would read like a *Who's Who of the World*, from art to politics. Sarah Bernhardt and her Italian counterpart Eleonora Duse used the train to thrill the stages of Europe. For musicians there were Toscanini and Mahler. Dancers Nijinsky and Pavlova were there, while lesser performers like Harry Houdini and the girls of the Ziegfeld Follies also rode the rails. Violinists were allowed to practice on the train, and occasionally one might see trapeze artists hanging like bats from the baggage racks.
>
> — Barnaby Conrad III, "Train of Kings"

If a sentence does not support the topic sentence directly, readers expect it to support another sentence in the paragraph. The following paragraph begins with a topic sentence. The italicized sentences are direct supports, and the rest of the sentences are indirect supports.

> Though the open-space classroom works for many children, it is not practical for my son, David. *First, David is hyperactive.* When he was placed in an open-space classroom, he became distracted and confused. He was tempted to watch the movement going on around him instead of concentrating on his own work. *Second, David has a tendency to transpose letters and numbers, a tendency that can be overcome only by individual attention from the instructor.* In the open classroom he was moved from teacher to teacher, with each one responsible for a different subject. No single teacher worked with David long enough to diagnose the problem, let alone help him with it. *Finally, David is not a highly motivated learner.* In the open classroom, he was graded "at his own level," not by criteria for a certain grade. He could receive a B in reading and still be a grade level behind, because he was doing satisfactory work "at his own level." [Italics added.]
>
> — Margaret Smith, student

Repeating key words

Repetition of key words is an important technique for gaining coherence. To prevent repetitions from becoming dull, you can use variations of the key word (*hike, hiker, hiking*), pronouns referring to the word (*gamblers . . . they*), and synonyms (*run, spring, race, dash*). In the following paragraph describing plots among indentured servants in the seventeenth century, historian Richard Hofstadter binds sentences together by repeating the key word *plots* and echoing it with variations (italicized).

> *Plots* hatched by several servants to run away together occurred mostly in the plantation colonies, and the few recorded servant *uprisings* were entirely limited to those colonies. Virginia had been forced from its very earliest years to take stringent steps against *mutinous plots*, and severe punishments for *such behavior* were recorded. Most servant *plots* occurred in the seventeenth century: a contemplated *uprising* was nipped in the bud in York County in 1661; apparently led by some left-wing offshoots of the *Great Rebellion*, servants *plotted* an *insurrection* in Gloucester County in 1663, and four leaders were condemned and executed; some discontented servants apparently joined *Bacon's Rebellion* in the 1670's. In the 1680's the planters became newly apprehensive of discontent among the servants "owing to their great necessities and want of clothes," and it was feared they would *rise up* and *plunder* the storehouses and ships; in 1682 there were plant-cutting *riots* in which servants and laborers, as well as some planters, took part. [Italics added.]
>
> — Richard Hofstadter, *America at 1750*

Using parallel structures

Parallel structures are frequently used within sentences to underscore the similarity of ideas (see S1). They may also be used to bind together a series of sentences expressing similar information. In the following passage describing folk beliefs, anthropologist Margaret Mead presents similar information in parallel grammatical form.

> Actually, almost every day, even in the most sophisticated home, something is likely to happen that evokes the memory of some old folk belief. The salt spills. A knife falls to the floor. Your nose tickles. Then perhaps, with a slightly embarrassed smile, the person who spilled the salt tosses a pinch over his left shoulder. Or someone recites the old rhyme, "Knife falls, gentleman calls." Or as you rub your nose you think, That means a letter. I wonder who's writing?   — Margaret Mead, "New Superstitions for Old"

Maintaining consistency

Coherence suffers whenever a draft shifts confusingly from one point of view to another (for example, from *I* to *you* or from *anyone* to *they*). Coherence also suffers when a draft shifts without reason from one verb tense to another (for example, from *swam* to *swims*). For advice on avoiding shifts, see S4.

Providing transitions

Transitions are bridges between what has been read and what is about to be read. Transitions help readers move from sentence to sentence; they also alert readers to more global connections of ideas — those between paragraphs or even larger blocks of text.

ACADEMIC ENGLISH Choose transitions carefully and vary them appropriately. For instance, avoid using a transition that signals a logical relationship (such as *therefore*) if no clear logical relationship exists. Each transition has a different meaning; if you do not use an appropriate signal, you might confuse your reader.

▶ Although taking eight o'clock classes may seem unappealing,

                                               For example,

  coming to school early has its advantages. ~~Moreover,~~

  students who arrive early typically avoid the worst traffic

  and find the best parking spaces.

SENTENCE-LEVEL TRANSITIONS Certain words and phrases signal connections between (or within) sentences. Frequently used transitions are included in the chart on page 36.

Skilled writers use transitional expressions with care, making sure, for example, not to use *consequently* when *also* would be more precise. They are also careful to select transitions with an appropriate tone, perhaps preferring *so* to *thus* in an informal piece, *in summary* to *in short* for a scholarly essay.

In the following paragraph, taken from an argument that dinosaurs had the "'right-sized' brains for reptiles of their body size," biologist Stephen Jay Gould uses transitions (italicized) with skill.

I don't wish to deny that the flattened, minuscule head of largebodied *Stegosaurus* houses little brain from our subjective, top-heavy perspective, *but* I do wish to assert that we should not expect more of the beast. *First of all*, large animals have relatively smaller brains than related, small animals. The correlation of brain size with body size among kindred animals (all reptiles, all mammals, *for example*) is remarkably regular. *As* we move from small to large animals, from mice to elephants or small lizards to Komodo dragons, brain size increases, *but* not so fast as body size. *In other words*, bodies grow faster than brains, *and* large animals have low ratios of brain weight to body weight. *In fact*, brains grow only about two-thirds as fast as bodies. *Since* we have no reason to believe that large animals are consistently stupider than their smaller relatives, we must conclude that large animals require relatively less brain to do as well as smaller animals. *If* we do not recognize this relationship, we are likely to underestimate the mental power of very large animals, dinosaurs *in particular.*

— Stephen Jay Gould, "Were Dinosaurs Dumb?"

ON THE WEB > dianahacker.com/writersref
Writing exercises > E-ex C4–2

PARAGRAPH-LEVEL TRANSITIONS Transitions between paragraphs usually link the *first* sentence of a new paragraph with the *first* sentence of the previous paragraph. In other words, the topic sentences signal global connections.

Look for opportunities to allude to the subject of a previous paragraph (as summed up in its topic sentence) in the topic sentence of the next paragraph. In his essay "Little Green Lies," Jonathan H. Alder uses this strategy in the following topic sentences, which appear in a passage describing the benefits of plastic packaging.

Consider aseptic packaging, the synthetic packaging for the "juice boxes" so many children bring to school with their lunch. One criticism of aseptic packaging is that it is nearly impossible to recycle, yet on almost every other count, aseptic packaging is environmentally preferable to the packaging alternatives. Not only do aseptic containers not require refrigeration to keep their contents from spoiling, but their manufacture requires less than one-10th the energy of making glass bottles.

What is true for juice boxes is also true for other forms of synthetic packaging. The use of polystyrene, which is commonly (and mistakenly) referred to as "Styrofoam," can reduce food waste dramatically due to its insulating properties. (Thanks to these properties, polystyrene cups are much preferred over paper for that morning cup of coffee.) Polystyrene also requires significantly fewer resources to produce than its paper counterpart.

TRANSITIONS BETWEEN BLOCKS OF TEXT In long essays, you may need to alert readers to connections between large blocks of text. You can do this by inserting transitional paragraphs at key points in the essay. On the next page, for example, is a transitional paragraph from a student research paper. It announces that the first part of the paper has come to a close and the second part is about to begin.

Common transitions

TO SHOW ADDITION and, also, besides, further, furthermore, in addition, moreover, next, too, first, second

TO GIVE EXAMPLES for example, for instance, to illustrate, in fact, specifically

TO COMPARE also, in the same manner, similarly, likewise

TO CONTRAST but, however, on the other hand, in contrast, nevertheless, still, even though, on the contrary, yet, although

TO SUMMARIZE OR CONCLUDE in other words, in short, in summary, in conclusion, to sum up, that is, therefore

TO SHOW TIME after, as, before, next, during, later, finally, meanwhile, since, then, when, while, immediately

TO SHOW PLACE OR DIRECTION above, below, beyond, farther on, nearby, opposite, close, to the left

TO INDICATE LOGICAL RELATIONSHIP if, so, therefore, consequently, thus, as a result, for this reason, because, since

> Although the great apes have demonstrated significant language skills, one central question remains: Can they be taught to use that uniquely human language tool we call grammar, to learn the difference, for instance, between "ape bite human" and "human bite ape"? In other words, can an ape create a sentence?

C4-e If necessary, adjust paragraph length.

Most readers feel comfortable reading paragraphs that range between one hundred and two hundred words. Shorter paragraphs force too much starting and stopping, and longer ones strain the reader's attention span. There are exceptions to this guideline, however. Paragraphs longer than two hundred words frequently appear in scholarly writing, where they suggest seriousness and depth. Paragraphs shorter than one hundred words occur in newspapers because of narrow columns; in informal essays to quicken the pace; in business letters, where readers routinely skim for main ideas; and in e-mail and on Web sites for ease of reading on the computer screen.

In an essay, the first and last paragraphs will ordinarily be the introduction and conclusion. These special-purpose paragraphs are likely to be shorter than the paragraphs in the body of the essay.

Typically, the body paragraphs will follow the essay's outline: one paragraph per point in short essays, a group of paragraphs per point in longer ones. Some ideas require more development than others, however, so it is best to be flexible. If an idea stretches to a length unreasonable for a paragraph, you should divide the paragraph, even if you have presented comparable points in the essay in single paragraphs.

Paragraph breaks are not always made for strictly logical reasons. Writers use them for all of the following reasons.

REASONS FOR BEGINNING A NEW PARAGRAPH

- to mark off the introduction and the conclusion
- to signal a shift to a new idea
- to indicate an important shift in time or place
- to emphasize a point (by placing it at the beginning or the end, not in the middle, of a paragraph)
- to highlight a contrast
- to signal a change of speakers (in dialogue)
- to provide readers with a needed pause
- to break up text that looks too dense

Beware of using too many short, choppy paragraphs, however. Readers want to see how your ideas connect, and they become irritated when you break their momentum by forcing them to pause every few sentences. Here are some reasons you might have for combining some of the paragraphs in a rough draft.

REASONS FOR COMBINING PARAGRAPHS

- to clarify the essay's organization
- to connect closely related ideas
- to bind together text that looks too choppy

C5

Designing documents

The term *document* is broad enough to describe anything you might write in a college class, in the business world, and in everyday life. How you design a document (format it for the printed page or for a computer screen) will affect how readers respond to it.

Good document design promotes readability, but what *readability* means depends on your purpose and audience and perhaps on other elements of your writing situation, such as your subject and any length restrictions. All of your design choices — layout, word processing options such as margins and fonts, headings, and lists — should be made in light of your writing situation. Likewise, different types of visuals — tables, charts, and images — can support your writing if they are used appropriately.

C5-a Determine layout and format to suit your purpose and audience.

Word processing programs offer abundant options for layout, margins and line spacing, alignment, and fonts. As you use these options to design documents, always keep the purpose of the document and the needs of your readers in mind.

Layout

Most readers have set ideas about how different kinds of documents should look. Advertisements, for example, have a distinctive appearance, as do newsletters, flyers, brochures, and menus. Instructors have expectations about how a college paper should look (see C5-e). Employers expect documents such as letters, résumés, and memos to be presented in standard ways (see C5-f). And anyone who reads your writing online will appreciate a recognizable layout.

Unless you have a compelling reason to stray from convention, it's best to choose a document layout that conforms to your readers' expectations. If you're not sure what readers expect, look at examples of the kind of document you are producing.

Planning a document: Purpose and audience checklist

- What is the purpose of your document? How can your document design help you achieve this purpose?
- Who are your readers? What are their expectations?
- What format is required? What format options — layout, margins, line spacing, alignment, and fonts — will readers expect?
- How can you use visuals — charts, graphs, tables, images — to help you convey information?

Margins and line spacing

Margins help control the look of a page. For most academic and business documents, leave a margin of one to one and a half inches on all sides. These margins create a visual frame for the text and provide room for annotations, such as an instructor's comments or a co-worker's suggestions. Narrower margins generally make a page crowded and difficult to read.

SINGLE-SPACED, UNFORMATTED

Obesity in Children   1

Can Medication Cure Obesity in Children?
A Review of the Literature

In March 2004, U.S. Surgeon General Richard Carmona called attention to a health problem in the United States that, until recently, has been overlooked: childhood obesity. Carmona said that the "astounding" 15% child obesity rate constitutes an "epidemic." Since the early 1980s, that rate has "doubled in children and tripled in adolescents." Now more than 9 million children are classified as obese (paras. 3, 6). While the traditional response to a medical epidemic is to hunt for a vaccine or a cure-all pill, childhood obesity has proven more elusive. The lack of success of recent initiatives suggests that medication might not be the answer for the escalating problem. This literature review considers whether the use of medication is a promising approach for solving the childhood obesity problem by responding to the following questions: What are the implications of childhood obesity? Is medication effective at treating childhood obesity? Is medication safe for children? Is medication the best solution? Understanding the limitations of medical treatments for children highlights the complexity of the childhood obesity problem in the United States and underscores the need for physicians, advocacy groups, and policymakers to search for other solutions.

Obesity can be a devastating problem from both an individual and a societal perspective. Obesity puts children at risk for a number of medical complications, including type 2 diabetes, hypertension, sleep apnea, and orthopedic problems (Henry J. Kaiser Family Foundation, 2004, p. 1). Researchers Hoppin and Taveras (2004) have noted that obesity is often associated with psychological issues such as depression, anxiety, and binge eating (Table 4).

Obesity also poses serious problems for a society struggling to cope with rising health care costs. The cost of treating obesity currently totals $117 billion per year--a price, according to the surgeon general, "second only to the cost of [treating] tobacco use" (Carmona, 2004, para. 9). And as the number of children who suffer from obesity grows, long-term costs will only increase.

The widening scope of the obesity problem has prompted medical professionals to rethink old conceptions of the disorder and its causes. As researchers Yanovski and Yanovski (2002) have explained, obesity

DOUBLE-SPACED, FORMATTED

Obesity in Children   1

Can Medication Cure Obesity in Children?
A Review of the Literature

In March 2004, U.S. Surgeon General Richard Carmona called attention to a health problem in the United States that, until recently, has been overlooked: childhood obesity. Carmona said that the "astounding" 15% child obesity rate constitutes an "epidemic." Since the early 1980s, that rate has "doubled in children and tripled in adolescents." Now more than 9 million children are classified as obese (paras. 3, 6).[1] While the traditional response to a medical epidemic is to hunt for a vaccine or a cure-all pill, childhood obesity has proven more elusive. The lack of success of recent initiatives suggests that medication might not be the answer for the escalating problem. This literature review considers whether the use of medication is a promising approach for solving the childhood obesity problem by responding to the following questions:

1. What are the implications of childhood obesity?
2. Is medication effective at treating childhood obesity?
3. Is medication safe for children?
4. Is medication the best solution?

Understanding the limitations of medical treatments for children highlights the complexity of the childhood obesity

[1]Obesity is measured in terms of body-mass index (BMI): weight in kilograms divided by square of height in meters. An adult with a BMI 30 or higher is considered obese. In children and adolescents, obesity is defined in relation to others of the same age and gender. An adolescent with a BMI in the 95th percentile for his or her age and gender is considered obese.

ACADEMIC ENGLISH   If your word processing program was not purchased in the United States, you may need to change the default settings. From your page setup menu (usually under the file menu) change the paper size to 8.5×11 inches (21.5×28 cm). In most cases, change your margins to one inch (2.5 or 2.6 cm).

Most manuscripts in progress are double-spaced to allow room for editing. Final copy is often double-spaced as well, since single-spacing is less inviting to read. If you are unsure about margin and spacing requirements, check with your instructor or look at documents similar to the one you are writing. At times, the advantages of double-spacing are offset by other considerations. For example, most business and technical documents are single-spaced, with double-spacing between paragraphs, to save paper and to promote quick scanning. Your document's purpose and context should determine appropriate margins and line spacing.

Alignment

Word processing programs allow you to align text and visuals on a page in four ways: left, right, centered, and justified. Most academic and business documents are left-aligned for easy reading. Although justified margins may seem more professional, they tend to create awkward word spacing and should be avoided.

Fonts

If you have a choice, select a font that fits your writing situation in an easy-to-read size (usually 10–12 points). Although offbeat or decorative fonts, such as those that look handwritten, may seem attractive, they slow readers down and can distract them from your ideas. For example, using comic sans, a font with a handwritten, childish feel, can make an essay seem too informal or unpolished, regardless of how well it is written. Fonts that are easy to read and appropriate for college and workplace documents include the following:

Arial	Tahoma
Courier	Times New Roman
Garamond	Verdana
Georgia	

Font styles — such as **boldface**, *italics*, and underlining — can be useful for calling attention to parts of a document. On the whole, it is best to use restraint when selecting font styles. Applying too many different styles within a document results in busy-looking pages and confuses readers.

TIP: Never write a document in all capital or all lowercase letters. Doing so can frustrate or annoy readers. Although some readers have become accustomed to e-mails that omit capital letters entirely, their absence makes a message difficult to read.

ON THE WEB > dianahacker.com/writersref
Links Library > Document design

C5-b Use headings when appropriate.

You will have little need for headings in short essays, especially if you use paragraphing and clear topic sentences to guide readers. In more complex documents, however, such as research papers, grant proposals, business reports, and Web sites, headings can be a useful visual cue for readers.

Headings help readers see at a glance the organization of a document. If more than one level of heading is used, the headings also indicate the hierarchy of ideas — as they do throughout this book.

Headings can serve a number of functions for your readers. When readers are simply looking up information, headings will help them find it quickly. When readers are scanning, hoping to pick up the gist of things, headings will guide them. Even when readers are committed enough to read every word, headings can help. Efficient readers preview a document before they begin reading; when previewing and while reading, they are guided by any visual cues the writer provides.

TIP: While headings can be useful, they cannot substitute for transitions between paragraphs. Keep this in mind as you write college essays.

Phrasing headings

Headings should be as brief and as informative as possible. Certain styles of headings — the most common being -*ing* phrases, noun phrases, questions, and imperative sentences — work better for some purposes, audiences, and subjects than others.

Whatever style you choose, use it consistently. Headings on the same level of organization should be written in parallel structure (see S1), as in the following examples from a report, a history textbook, a financial brochure, and a nursing manual, respectively.

-*ING* HEADINGS

Safeguarding the earth's atmosphere

Charting the path to sustainable energy

Conserving global forests

NOUN PHRASE HEADINGS

The economics of slavery

The sociology of slavery

The psychological effects of slavery

QUESTIONS AS HEADINGS

How do I buy shares?

How do I redeem shares?

What is the history of the fund's performance?

IMPERATIVE SENTENCES AS HEADINGS

Ask the patient to describe current symptoms.

Take a detailed medical history.

Record the patient's vital signs.

Placing and formatting headings

Headings on the same level of organization should be placed and formatted in a consistent way. If you have more than one level of heading, you might center your first-level headings and make them boldface; then you might make the second-level headings left-aligned and italicized, like this:

First-level heading

Second-level heading

A college paper with headings typically has only one level, and the headings are often centered, as in the sample paper on pages 484–88. Business memos often include headings. Important headings can be highlighted by using white space around them. Less important headings can be downplayed by using less white space or by running them into the text.

C5-c Use lists to guide readers.

Lists are easy to read or scan when they are displayed rather than run into your text. You might choose to display the following kinds of lists:

- steps in a process
- materials needed for a project
- parts of an object
- advice or recommendations
- items to be discussed
- criteria for evaluation (as in checklists)

Lists should usually be introduced with an independent clause followed by a colon (*All mammals share the following five characteristics:*). Periods are not used after items in a list unless the items are complete sentences.

If the order of items is not important, use bullets (circles or squares) or dashes to draw readers' eyes to a list. If you are describing a sequence or a set of steps, number the list with arabic numerals (1, 2, 3) followed by periods.

TIP: Although lists can be useful visual cues, don't overdo them. Too many will clutter a document.

C5-d Add visuals to supplement your text.

Visuals can convey information concisely and powerfully. Charts, graphs, and tables, for example, can simplify complex numerical data. Images — including photographs and diagrams — often express an idea more vividly than words can. With access to the Internet, digital photography, and word processing or desktop publishing software, you can download or create your own visuals to enhance your document. If you download a visual, you must credit your source (see R3).

Choosing appropriate visuals

Use visuals to supplement your writing, not to substitute for it. Always consider how a visual supports your purpose and how your audience might respond to it. A student writing about electronic surveillance in the workplace, for example, used a cartoon to illustrate her point about employees' personal use of the Internet at work (see MLA-5b). Another student, writing about treatments for childhood obesity, created a table to display data she had found in two different sources and discussed in her paper (see APA-5b).

As you draft and revise a document, choose carefully the visuals that support your main point, and avoid overloading your text with too many images. The chart on pages 44–45 describes eight types of visuals and their purposes.

Placing and labeling visuals

A visual may be placed in the text of a document, near a discussion to which it relates, or it can be put in an appendix, labeled, and referred to in the text.

Choosing visuals to suit your purpose

Pie chart
Pie charts compare a part or parts to the whole. The parts are displayed as segments of the pie, represented as percentages of the whole (which is always 100 percent).

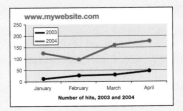

Use of the George Mason University writing center, by group, academic year 2003–04

■ Juniors 30%
▥ Seniors 20%
■ First-year students 17%
▢ Sophomores 17%
■ Graduate students 11%
▨ Not indicated 3%
■ Staff / alumni 2%

Line graph
Line graphs highlight trends over a period of time or compare numerical data.

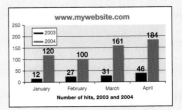

www.mywebsite.com

— 2003
— 2004

January February March April

Number of hits, 2003 and 2004

Bar graph
Bar graphs can be used for the same purpose as line graphs. This bar graph displays the same data as in the line graph above.

www.mywebsite.com

— 2003
— 2004

	January	February	March	April
2004	120	100	161	184
2003	12	27	31	46

Number of hits, 2003 and 2004

Table
Tables organize complicated numerical information into an accessible format.

Prices of daily doses of AIDS drugs ($US)

Drug	Brazil	Uganda	Côte d'Ivoire	US
3TC (Lamuvidine)	1.66	3.28	2.95	8.70
ddC (Zalcitabine)	0.24	4.17	3.75	8.80
Didanosine	2.04	5.26	3.48	7.25
Efavirenz	6.96	n/a	6.41	13.13
Indinavir	10.32	12.79	9.07	14.93
Nelfinavir	4.14	4.45	4.39	6.47
Nevirapine	5.04	n/a	n/a	8.48
Saquinavir	6.24	7.37	5.52	8.50
Stavudine	0.56	6.19	4.10	9.07
ZDV/3TC	1.44	7.34	n/a	18.78
Zidovudine	1.08	4.34	2.43	10.12

Source: UNAIDS, 2000

Photograph

Photographs vividly depict people, scenes, or objects discussed in a text.

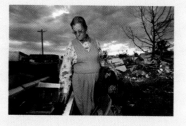

Diagram

Diagrams, useful in scientific and technical writing, concisely illustrate processes, structures, or interactions.

Map

Maps indicate locations, distances, and demographic information.

Flowchart

Flowcharts show structures or steps in a process. (For another example, see p. 104.)

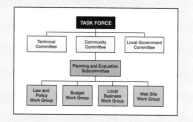

VISUAL WITH A SOURCE CREDITED

Fig. 6.

Postal Service Size, by Number of Employees

	Among the Global 500			Among US Companies	
Rank	Company	Employees as of 2002	Rank	Company	Employees as of 2002
1	Wal-Mart Stores	1,300,000	1	Wal-Mart Stores	1,300,000
2	China National Petroleum	1,146,194	**2**	**US Postal Service**	**854,376**
3	Sinopec	917,000	3	McDonald's	413,000
4	**US Postal Service**	**854,376**	4	United Parcel Service	360,000
5	Agricultural Bank of China	490,999	5	Ford Motor	350,321
6	Siemens	426,000	6	General Motors	350,000
7	McDonald's	413,000	7	Intl. Business Machines	315,889
8	Ind. & Comm. Bank of China	405,000	8	General Electric	315,000
9	Carrefour	396,662	9	Target	306,000
10	Compass Group	392,352	10	Home Depot	300,000
11	China Telecomm	365,778	11	Kroger	289,000
12	DaimlerChrysler	365,571	12	Sears Roebuck	289,000
13	United Parcel Service	360,000	13	Tyco International	267,000
14	Ford Motor	350,321	14	Citigroup	252,500
15	General Motors	350,000	15	Verizon Communications	229,497

Source: Number of employees rankings by *Fortune Magazine,* April 14, 2003.

Placing visuals in the text of a document can be tricky. Usually you will want the visual to appear close to the sentences that relate to it, but page breaks won't always allow this placement. At times you may need to insert the visual at a later point and tell readers where it can be found; sometimes, with the help of software, you can make the text flow around the visual. No matter where you place a visual, refer to it in your text. Don't expect visuals to speak for themselves.

Most of the visuals you include in a document will require some sort of label. Labels, which are typically placed above or under the visuals, should be brief but descriptive. Most commonly, a visual is labeled with the word "Figure" or the abbreviation "Fig.," followed by a number: *Fig. 4.* Sometimes a title might be included to explain how the visual relates to the text: *Fig. 4. Voter turnout by age.*

Using visuals responsibly

Most word processing and spreadsheet software will allow you to produce your own visuals. If you create a chart, a table, or a graph using information from your research, you must cite the source of the information even though the visual is your own. The table on page 46 credits the source of its data.

If you download a photograph from the Web or scan an image from a magazine or book, you must credit the person or organization that created it, just as you would cite any other source you use in a college paper (see R3). If your document is written for publication outside the classroom, you will need to request permission to use any visual you borrow.

Guidelines for using visuals vary by academic discipline. See MLA-5a, APA-5a, and CMS-5a for guidelines in English and humanities, social sciences, and history, respectively.

C5-e Use standard academic formatting.

Instructors have certain expectations about how a college paper should look. If your instructor provides guidelines for formatting an essay, report, or research paper, you should follow them. Otherwise, use the manuscript format that is recommended for your academic discipline.

In most English and humanities classes, you will be asked to use the MLA (Modern Language Association) format. The sample on pages 48–49 illustrates this format. For more detailed MLA manuscript guidelines and a sample research paper, see MLA-5. If you have been asked to use APA (American Psychological Association) or CMS (*Chicago Manual of Style*) manuscript guidelines, see APA-5 or CMS-5.

MLA ESSAY FORMAT

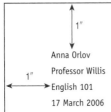

1/2″

Orlov 1

1″

Anna Orlov

1″ Professor Willis

English 101

17 March 2006

Title is centered.

Online Monitoring:

1/2″ A Threat to Employee Privacy in the Wired Workplace

As the Internet has become an integral tool of businesses, company policies on Internet usage have become as common as policies regarding vacation days or sexual harassment. A 2005 study by the American Management Association and ePolicy Institute found that 76% of

Double-spacing is used throughout.

companies monitor employees' use of the Web, and the number of companies that block employees' access to certain Web sites has increased 1″ 27% since 2001 (1). Unlike other company rules, however, Internet usage policies often include language authorizing companies to secretly monitor their employees, a practice that raises questions about rights in the workplace. Although companies often have legitimate concerns that lead them to monitor employees' Internet usage--from expensive security breaches to reduced productivity--the benefits of electronic surveillance are outweighed by its costs to employees' privacy and autonomy.

While surveillance of employees is not a new phenomenon, electronic surveillance allows employers to monitor workers with unprecedented efficiency. In his book The Naked Employee, Frederick Lane describes offline ways in which employers have been permitted to intrude on employees' privacy for decades, such as drug testing, background checks, psychological exams, lie detector tests, and in-store video surveillance. The difference, Lane argues, between these old methods of data gathering and electronic surveillance involves quantity:

Technology makes it possible for employers to gather 1″ enormous amounts of data about employees, often far beyond what is necessary to satisfy safety or productivity concerns. And the trends that drive technology--faster, smaller, cheaper--make it possible for larger and larger numbers of employers to gather ever-greater amounts of personal data. (3-4)

1″

Marginal annotations indicate MLA-style formatting.

MLA ESSAY FORMAT (*continued*)

½″
1″
Orlov 5

Works Cited · Heading is centered.

Adams, Scott. Dilbert and the Way of the Weasel. New York: Harper,
2002.

American Management Association and ePolicy Institute. "2005
Electronic Monitoring and Surveillance Survey."
American Management Association. 2005. 15 Feb. 2006
<http://www.amanet.org/research/pdfs/
EMS_summary05.pdf>.

"Automatically Record Everything They Do Online! Spector Pro 5.0
FAQ's." Netbus.org. SpectorSoft. 17 Feb. 2006 <http://
www.netbus.org/sProFAQ.html>.

1″ ← Flynn, Nancy. "Internet Policies." ePolicy Institute. 2001. 15
Feb. 2006 <http://www.epolicyinstitute.com/i_policies/
index.html>.

Frauenheim, Ed. "Stop Reading This Headline and Get Back to Work." ← 1″ →
½″ ← CNET News.com. 11 July 2005. 17 Feb. 2006 <http://
news.com/Stop+reading+this+headline+and+get+
back+to+work/2100-1022_3-5783552.html>.

Gonsalves, Chris. "Wasting Away on the Web." eWeek.com 8 Aug. · Double-spacing is
2005. 16 Feb. 2006 <http://www.eweek.com/article2/ · used throughout.;
0,1895,1843242,00.asp>. · no extra space
between entries.

Kesan, Jay P. "Cyber-Working or Cyber-Shirking? A First Principles
Examination of Electronic Privacy in the Workplace." Florida Law
Review 54 (2002): 289-332.

Lane, Frederick S., III. The Naked Employee: How Technology Is
Compromising Workplace Privacy. New York: Amer. Management
Assn., 2003.

Tam, Pui-Wing, et al. "Snooping E-Mail by Software Is Now a
Workplace Norm." Wall Street Journal 9 Mar. 2005: B1+.

Tynan, Daniel. "Your Boss Is Watching." PC World 6 Oct. 2004. 17 Feb.
2006 <http://www.pcworld.com/news/article/0,aid,118072,00.asp>.

Verespej, Michael A. "Inappropriate Internet Surfing." Industry Week
7 Feb. 2000. 16 Feb. 2006 <http://www.industryweek.com/
ReadArticle.aspx?ArticleID=568>.

C5-f Use standard business formatting.

This section provides advice on preparing business letters, résumés, and memos. For a more detailed discussion of these and other business documents — proposals, reports, executive summaries, and so on — consult a business writing textbook or look at current examples at the organization for which you are writing.

ON THE WEB > dianahacker.com/writersref
Links Library > Document design

BUSINESS LETTER IN FULL BLOCK STYLE

LatinoVoice

March 16, 2005 ——— Date

Jonathan Ross
Managing Editor
Latino World Today   Inside
2971 East Oak Avenue   address
Baltimore, MD 21201

Dear Mr. Ross: ——— Salutation

Thank you very much for taking the time yesterday to speak to the University of Maryland's Latino Club. A number of students have told me that they enjoyed your presentation and found your job search suggestions to be extremely helpful.

As I mentioned to you when we first scheduled your appearance, the club publishes a monthly newsletter, *Latino Voice.* Our purpose is to share up-to-date information and expert advice with members of the university's Latino population. Considering how much students benefited from your talk, I would like to publish excerpts from it in our newsletter.

Body — I have taken the liberty of transcribing parts of your presentation and organizing them into a question-and-answer format for our readers. When you have a moment, would you mind looking through the enclosed article and letting me know if I may have your permission to print it? I would be happy, of course, to make any changes or corrections that you request. I'm hoping to include this article in our next newsletter, so I would need your response by April 4.

Once again, Mr. Ross, thank you for sharing your experiences with us. You gave an informative and entertaining speech, and I would love to be able to share it with the students who couldn't hear it in person.

Sincerely, ——— Close

Jeffrey Richardson

Jeffrey Richardson   Signature
Associate Editor

Enc.

210 Student Center University of Maryland College Park MD 20742

Business letters

In writing a business letter, be direct, clear, and courteous. State your purpose or request at the beginning of the letter and include only relevant information in the body. Being as direct and concise as possible shows that you value your reader's time. For the format of the letter, stick to established business conventions. A sample business letter in *full block* style appears on page 50.

Résumés and cover letters

An effective résumé gives relevant information in a clear, concise form. You may be asked to produce a traditional résumé, a scannable résumé, or a Web résumé. A cover letter gives a prospective employer a reason to look at your résumé. The goal is to present yourself in a favorable light without including unnecessary details and wasting your reader's time.

COVER LETTERS When you send out your résumé, always include a cover letter that introduces yourself, states the position you seek, and tells where you learned about it. The letter should also highlight past experiences that qualify you for the position and emphasize what you can do for the employer (not what the job will do for you). End the letter with a suggestion for a meeting, and tell your prospective employer when you will be available.

TRADITIONAL RÉSUMÉS Traditional paper résumés are screened by people, not by computers. Because screeners may face stacks of applications, they often spend very little time looking at each résumé. Therefore, you will need to make your résumé as reader-friendly as possible. Here are a few guidelines. See page 52 for an example.

- Limit your résumé to one page if possible, two pages at the most.
- Organize your information into clear categories — Education, Experience, and so on.
- Present the information in each category in reverse chronological order to highlight your most recent accomplishments.
- Use bulleted lists or some other simple, clear visual device to organize information.
- Use strong, active verbs to emphasize your accomplishments. (Use present-tense verbs, such as *manage,* for current activities and past-tense verbs, such as *managed,* for past activities.)

TRADITIONAL RÉSUMÉ

Jeffrey Richardson

121 Knox Road, #6
College Park, MD 20740
301–555–2651
jrichardson@jrichardson.localhost

OBJECTIVE

To obtain an editorial internship with a magazine

EDUCATION

Fall 2002 –
present

University of Maryland
• BA expected in June 2006
• Double major: English and Latin American studies
• GPA: 3.7 (on a 4-point scale)

EXPERIENCE

Fall 2004 –
present

Associate editor, *Latino Voice*, newsletter of Latino Club
• Assign and edit feature articles
• Coordinate community outreach

Fall 2003 –
present

Photo editor, *The Diamondback*, college paper
• Shoot and print photographs
• Select and lay out photographs and other visuals

Summer 2004

Intern, *The Globe,* Fairfax, Virginia
• Wrote stories about local issues and personalities
• Interviewed political candidates
• Edited and proofread copy
• Coedited "The Landscapes of Northern Virginia:
  A Photoessay"

Summers
2003, 2004

Tutor, Fairfax County ESL Program
• Tutored Latino students in English as a Second Language
• Trained new tutors

ACTIVITIES

Photographers' Workshop, Latino Club

PORTFOLIO

Available at http://jrichardson.localhost/jrportfolio.htm

REFERENCES

Available upon request

SCANNABLE RÉSUMÉS   Scannable résumés might be submitted on paper, by e-mail, or through an online employment service. The prospective employer scans and searches the résumé electronically; a database matches keywords in the employer's job description with keywords in the résumé. A human screener then looks through the résumés filtered out by the database matching. A scannable résumé must be very simply formatted so that the scanner can accurately pick up its content. In general, follow these guidelines when preparing a scannable résumé:

- Include a Keywords section that lists words likely to be searched by a scanner. (Use nouns such as *manager*, not verbs such as *manage*.)

- Use standard résumé headings (Education, Experience, and so on).

- Avoid special characters, graphics, or font styles such as bold-face or italics.

WEB RÉSUMÉS   Posting your résumé on a Web site is an easy way to provide prospective employers with up-to-date information about your experience and employment goals. Web résumés allow you to present details about yourself without overwhelming your readers. Most guidelines for traditional résumés apply to Web résumés. Always list the date that you last updated the résumé.

ON THE WEB > dianahacker.com/writersref
Model papers > Résumés

Memos

Usually brief and to the point, a memo reports information, makes a request, or recommends an action. The format of a memo, which varies from company to company, is designed for easy distribution, quick reading, and efficient filing.

Most memos display the date, the name of the recipient, the name of the sender, and the subject on separate lines at the top of the page. Many companies have preprinted forms for memos, and some word processing programs allow you to call up a memo template.

The subject line of a memo, on paper or in e-mail, should describe the topic as clearly and concisely as possible, and the introductory paragraph should get right to the point. In addition, the body of the memo should be well organized and easy to skim. To promote skimming, use headings where possible and display any items that deserve special attention by setting them off from the text — in a list, for example, or in boldface.

E-mail

E-mail is fast replacing regular mail in the business world and in most people's personal lives. Especially in business and academic contexts, you will want to show readers that you value their time. Your message may be just one of many that your readers have to wade through. Here are some strategies for writing effective e-mails:

- Fill in the subject line with a meaningful, concise subject to help readers sort through messages and set priorities.

- Put the most important part of your message at the beginning so it will be seen on the first screen.

- For long, detailed messages, consider providing a summary at the beginning.

- Write concisely, and keep paragraphs fairly short, especially if your audience is likely to read your message on the screen.

- Avoid writing in all capital letters or all lowercase letters, a practice that is easy on the writer but hard on the reader.

- Use formatting such as boldface and italics and special characters sparingly; not all e-mail systems handle such elements consistently.

- Proofread for typos and obvious errors that are likely to slow down or annoy readers.

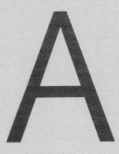

Academic Writing

A Academic Writing

Writing is a fact of college life. No matter what you study, you will be expected to participate in ongoing conversations conducted by other students and scholars. To join in those conversations, you will analyze and respond to texts, evaluate other people's arguments, and put forth your own ideas. Whatever the discipline, the goal of academic writing is to argue a thesis and support it with appropriate evidence.

A1

Writing about texts

The word *texts* can refer to a variety of works: essays, periodical articles, government reports, books, and even visuals such as advertisements and photographs. Most assignments that ask you to respond to a text call for a summary or an analysis or both.

A summary is neutral in tone and demonstrates that you have understood the author's key ideas. Assignments calling for an analysis of a text vary widely, but they will usually ask you to look at how the text's parts contribute to its central argument or purpose, often with the aim of judging its evidence or overall effect.

When you write about a written text, you will need to read it several times to digest its full meaning. Two techniques will help you move beyond a superficial first reading: (1) annotating the text with your observations and questions and (2) outlining the text's key points. The same techniques will help you analyze visual texts.

A1-a Read actively: Annotate the text.

Read actively by jotting down your questions, thoughts, and reactions in the margins of the text or in a notebook. Use a pencil instead of a highlighter; with a pencil you can underline key concepts, mark points, or circle elements that intrigue you. If you change your mind, you can erase your early annotations and replace them with new ones.

ON THE WEB > dianahacker.com/writersref
Resources for writers and tutors > Tips from writing tutors:
Benefits of reading

Guidelines for active reading

Familiarize yourself with the basic features and structure of a text.

- What kind of text are you reading? An essay? An editorial? A scholarly article? An advertisement? A photograph?
- What is the author's purpose? To inform? To persuade? To call to action?
- Who is the audience? How does the author attempt to appeal to the audience?
- What is the author's thesis? What question does the text attempt to answer?
- What evidence does the author provide to support the thesis?

Note details that surprise, puzzle, or intrigue you.

- Has the author revealed a fact or made a point that runs counter to what you had assumed was true? What exactly is surprising?
- Has the author made a generalization you disagree with? Can you think of evidence that would challenge the generalization?
- Are there any contradictions or inconsistencies in the text?
- Are there any words, statements, or phrases in the text that you don't understand? If so, what reference materials do you need to consult?

Read and reread to discover meaning.

- What do you notice on a second or third reading that you didn't notice earlier?
- Does the text raise questions that it does not resolve?
- If you could address the author directly, what questions would you pose? Where do you agree and disagree with the author? Why?

Apply critical thinking strategies to visual texts.

- What first strikes you about the image? What elements do you notice immediately?
- Who or what is the main subject of the image?
- What colors and textures dominate?
- What is in the background? In the foreground?
- What role, if any, do words play in the visual text?

Following are an article from a consumer-oriented newsletter and a magazine advertisement, annotated by students. The students, Emilia Sanchez and Albert Lee, were assigned to write a summary and an analysis. Each began by annotating the text.

ANNOTATED ARTICLE

Big Box Stores Are Bad for Main Street
BETSY TAYLOR

There is plenty of reason to be concerned about the proliferation of Wal-Marts and other so-called "big box" stores. The question, however, is not whether or not these types of stores create jobs (although several studies claim they produce a net job loss in local communities) or whether they ultimately save consumers money. The real concern about having a 25-acre slab of concrete with a 100,000 square foot box of stuff land on a town is whether it's good for a <u>community's soul.</u>

Opening strategy — the problem is not x, it's y.

Sentimental — what is a community's soul?

The worst thing about "big boxes" is that they have a tendency to produce Ross Perot's famous "big sucking sound" — sucking the life out of cities and small towns across the country. On the other hand, small businesses are great for a community. They offer more personal service; they won't threaten to pack up and leave town if they don't get tax breaks, free roads and other blandishments; and small-business owners are much more responsive to a customer's needs. (Ever try to complain about bad service or poor quality products <u>to the president</u> of Home Depot?)

Lumps all big boxes together.

Assumes all small businesses are attentive.

Logic problem? Why couldn't customer complain to store manager?

Yet, if big boxes are so bad, why are they so successful? One glaring reason is that (we've become a nation of hyperconsumers,) and the big-box boys know this. Downtown shopping districts comprised of small businesses take some of the efficiency out of overconsumption. There's all that hassle of having to travel from store to store, and having to pull out your credit card so many times. Occasionally, we even find ourselves chatting with the shopkeeper, wandering into a coffee shop to visit with a friend or otherwise wasting precious time that could be spent on acquiring more stuff.

True?

Nostalgia for a time that is long gone or never was.

But let's face it — bustling, thriving city centers are fun. They breathe life into a community. They allow cities and towns to stand out from each other. They provide an atmosphere for people to interact with each other that just cannot be found at Target, or Wal-Mart or Home Depot.

Community vs. economy. What about prices?

Is it anti-American to be against having a retail giant set up shop in one's community? Some people would say so. On the other hand, if you board up Main Street, what's left of America?

Ends with emotional appeal.

ANNOTATED ADVERTISEMENT

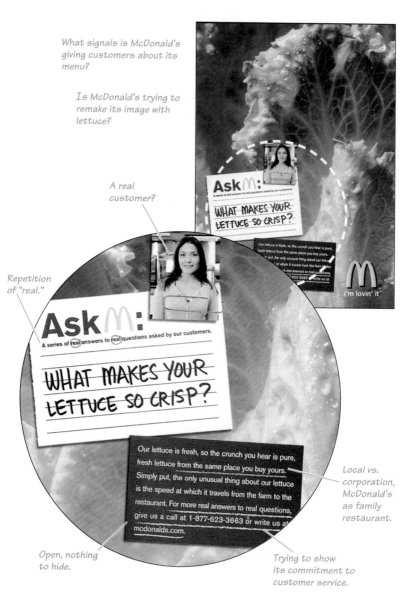

A1-b Try sketching a brief outline of the text.

After reading, rereading, and annotating a text, attempt to outline it. Seeing how the author has constructed a text can help you understand it. As you sketch an outline, pay special attention to the text's thesis (central idea) and its topic sentences. The thesis of a written text usually appears in the introduction, often in the first or second paragraph. Topic sentences can be found at the beginnings of most body paragraphs, where they announce a shift to a new topic. (See C2-a and C4-a.)

In your outline, put the author's thesis and key points in your own words. Here, for example, is the outline that Emilia Sanchez developed as she prepared to write her summary and analysis of the text printed on page 59. Notice that the outline does not simply trace the author's ideas paragraph by paragraph; instead, it sums up the article's central points.

OUTLINE OF "BIG BOX STORES ARE BAD FOR MAIN STREET"

Thesis: Whether or not they take jobs away from a community or offer low prices to consumers, we should be worried about "big-box" stores like Wal-Mart, Target, and Home Depot because they harm communities by taking the life out of downtown shopping districts.

I. Small businesses are better for cities and towns than big-box stores are.
   A. Small businesses offer personal service and big-box stores do not.
   B. Small businesses don't make demands on community resources as big-box stores do.
   C. Small businesses respond to customer concerns and big-box stores do not.
II. Big-box stores are successful because they cater to consumption at the expense of benefits to the community.
   A. Buying everything in one place is convenient.
   B. Shopping at small businesses may be inefficient, but it provides opportunities for socializing.
   C. Downtown shopping districts give each city or town a special identity.

Conclusion: While some people say that it's anti-American to oppose big-box stores, actually these stores threaten the communities that make up America by encouraging buying at the expense of the traditional interactions of Main Street.

A visual, of course, doesn't state an explicit thesis or an explicit line of reasoning. Instead, you must infer the meaning beneath the image's surface and interpret its central point and supporting ideas from the elements of its design. One way to outline a visual text is to try to define its purpose and sketch a list of its key elements. Here, for example, are the key features that Albert Lee identified for the advertisement printed on page 60.

Purpose: To persuade readers that McDonald's is concerned about its customers' health.

Key features:

- A close-up of a fresh, green lettuce leaf makes up the entire background.
- Near the center there's a comment card with a handwritten question from a "real" McDonald's customer: "What makes your lettuce so crisp?"
- A photograph of a smiling woman is clipped to the card.
- Beneath the comment card is the company's response, which emphasizes the farm-fresh quality and purity of its vegetables and urges customers to ask other candid questions.
- At the bottom of the ad is the McDonald's slogan "I'm lovin' it."

ON THE WEB > dianahacker.com/writersref
Model papers > Albert Lee

A1-c   Summarize to demonstrate your understanding.

Your goal in summarizing a text is to state the work's main ideas and key points simply, briefly, and accurately. If you have sketched a brief outline of the text (see A1-b), refer to it as you draft your summary.

To summarize a written text, first find the author's central idea — the thesis. Then divide the whole piece into a few major and perhaps minor ideas. Since a summary must be fairly short, you must make judgments about what is most important. To summarize a visual text, begin with information about who created the visual, who the intended audience is, and when and where the visual appeared. Briefly explain the visual's main point or purpose and point to its key features.

Following is Emilia Sanchez's summary of the article that is printed on page 59.

> In her essay "Big Box Stores Are Bad for Main Street," Betsy Taylor argues that chain stores harm communities by taking the life out of downtown shopping districts. Explaining that a commu-

Guidelines for writing a summary

- In the first sentence, mention the title of the text, the name of the author, and the author's thesis or the visual's central point.
- Maintain a neutral tone; be objective.
- Use the third-person point of view and the present tense.
- Keep your focus on the text. Don't state the author's ideas as if they were your own.
- Put all or most of your summary in your own words; if you borrow a phrase or a sentence from the text, put it in quotation marks and give the page number in parentheses.
- Limit yourself to presenting the text's key points.
- Be concise; make every word count.

nity's "soul" is more important than low prices or consumer convenience, she argues that small businesses are better than stores like Wal-Mart, Target, and Home Depot because they emphasize personal interactions and don't place demands on a community's resources. Taylor asserts that big-box stores are successful because "we've become a nation of hyper-consumers," although the convenience of shopping in these stores comes at the expense of benefits to the community. She concludes by suggesting that it's not "anti-American" to oppose big-box stores because the damage they inflict on downtown shopping districts extends to America itself.

— Emilia Sanchez, student

A1-d Analyze to demonstrate your critical thinking.

Whereas a summary most often answers the question of *what* a text says, an analysis looks at *how* a text makes its point.

Typically, an analysis takes the form of an essay that makes its own argument about a text. Include an introduction that briefly summarizes the text, a thesis that states your own judgment about the text, and body paragraphs that support your thesis with evidence. If you are analyzing an image, examine it as a whole and then reflect on how the individual elements contribute to its overall meaning. If you have written a summary of the text, you may find it useful to refer to the main points of the summary as you write your analysis.

Beginning on the next page is Emilia Sanchez's analysis of the article by Betsy Taylor (see p. 59).

Sanchez 1

Emilia Sanchez

Professor Goodwin

English 10

22 October 2005

Rethinking Big-Box Stores

Opening summarizes the article's purpose and thesis.

In her essay "Big Box Stores Are Bad for Main Street," Betsy Taylor focuses not on the economic effects of large chain stores but on the effects these stores have on the "soul" of America. She argues that stores like Home Depot, Target, and Wal-Mart are bad for America because they draw people out of downtown shopping districts and cause them to focus exclusively on consumption. In contrast, she believes that small businesses are good for America because they provide personal attention, foster community interaction, and make each city unique. But Taylor's argument is ultimately unconvincing because it is based on nostalgia--on idealized images of a quaint Main Street--rather than on the roles that businesses play in consumers' lives and communities. By ignoring the more complex, economically driven relationships between large chain stores and their communities, Taylor incorrectly assumes that simply getting rid of big-box stores would have a positive effect on America's communities.

Thesis expresses Sanchez's judgment of Taylor's article.

Taylor's use of colorful language reveals that she has a nostalgic view of American society and does not understand economic realities. In her first paragraph, Taylor refers to a big-box store as a "25-acre slab of concrete with a 100,000 square foot box of stuff" that "lands on a town," evoking images of a monolithic monster crushing the American way of life (1011). But her assessment oversimplifies a complex issue. Taylor does not consider that many downtown business districts failed long before chain stores moved in, when factories and mills closed and workers lost their jobs. In cities with struggling economies, big-box stores can actually provide much-needed jobs. Similarly, while Taylor blames big-box stores for harming local economies by asking for tax breaks, free roads, and other perks, she doesn't acknowledge that these stores also enter into economic partnerships with the surrounding communities by offering financial benefits to schools and hospitals.

Signal phrase introduces quotations from the source; Sanchez uses an MLA in-text citation.

Sanchez begins to identify and challenge Taylor's assumptions.

Marginal annotations indicate MLA-style formatting and effective writing.

Sanchez 2

Taylor's assumption that shopping in small businesses is always better for the customer also seems driven by nostalgia for an old-fashioned Main Street rather than by the facts. While she may be right that many small businesses offer personal service and are responsive to customer complaints, she does not consider that many customers appreciate the service at big-box stores. Just as customer service is better at some small businesses than at others, it is impossible to generalize about service at all big-box stores. For example, customers depend on the lenient return policies and the wide variety of products at stores like Target and Home Depot.

Taylor blames big-box stores for encouraging American "hyper-consumerism," but she oversimplifies by equating big-box stores with bad values and small businesses with good values. Like her other points, this claim ignores the economic and social realities of American society today. Big-box stores do not force Americans to buy more. By offering lower prices in a convenient setting, however, they allow consumers to save time and purchase goods they might not be able to afford from small businesses. The existence of more small businesses would not change what most Americans can afford, nor would it reduce their desire to buy affordable merchandise.

Taylor may be right that some big-box stores have a negative impact on communities and that small businesses offer certain advantages. But she ignores the economic conditions that support big-box stores as well as the fact that Main Street was in decline before the big-box store arrived. Getting rid of big-box stores will not bring back a simpler America populated by thriving, unique Main Streets; in reality, Main Street will not survive if consumers cannot afford to shop there.

Clear topic sentence announces a shift to a new topic.

Sanchez refutes Taylor's claim.

Sanchez treats the author fairly.

Conclusion returns to the thesis and shows the wider significance of Sanchez's analysis.

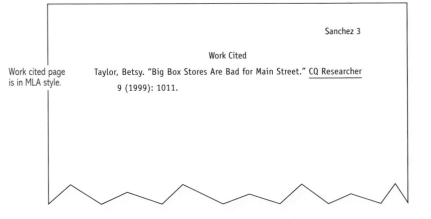

Work cited page is in MLA style.

Sanchez 3

Work Cited

Taylor, Betsy. "Big Box Stores Are Bad for Main Street." CQ Researcher 9 (1999): 1011.

Guidelines for analyzing a text

Written texts. Instructors who ask you to analyze a written nonfiction text often expect you to address some of the following questions.

- What is the author's thesis or central idea? Who is the audience?
- What questions does the author address (implicitly or explicitly)?
- How does the author structure the text? What are the key parts and how do they relate to one another and to the thesis?
- What strategies has the author used to generate interest in the argument and to persuade readers of its merit?
- What evidence does the author use to support the thesis? How persuasive is the evidence?
- Does the author anticipate objections and counter opposing views?
- Does the author fall prey to any faulty reasoning?

Visual texts. If you are analyzing a visual text, the following additional questions will help you evaluate an image's purpose and meaning.

- What surprises, perplexes, or intrigues you about the image?
- What clues suggest the visual text's intended audience? How does the image appeal to its audience?
- If the text is an advertisement, what product is it selling? Does it attempt to sell an idea or a message as well?
- If the visual text includes words, how do the words contribute to the meaning of the image?
- How do design elements — colors, shapes, perspective, background, foreground — shape the visual text's meaning or serve its purpose?

A2

Constructing reasonable arguments

In writing an argument, you take a stand on a debatable issue. The question being debated might be a matter of public policy:

> Should religious groups be allowed to meet on public school property?
> What is the least dangerous way to dispose of nuclear waste?
> Should a state enact laws rationing medical care?

On such questions, reasonable people may disagree.

Reasonable men and women also disagree about many scholarly issues. Psychologists debate the role of genes and environment in behavior; historians interpret causes of the Civil War quite differently; biologists challenge one another's predictions about the effects of global warming.

When you construct a *reasonable* argument, your goal is not simply to win or to have the last word. Your aim is to explain your understanding of the truth about a subject or to propose the best solution available for solving a problem — without being needlessly combative. In constructing your argument, you join a conversation with other writers and readers. Your aim is to convince readers to reconsider their opinions by offering new reasons to question an old viewpoint.

ACADEMIC ENGLISH Some cultures value writers who argue with force and express their superiority. Other cultures value writers who argue subtly or indirectly, often with an apology. Academic audiences in the United States will expect your writing to be assertive and confident — neither aggressive nor passive. Create an assertive tone by acknowledging different opinions and supporting your view with specific evidence.

TOO AGGRESSIVE Of course prayer should be discouraged in public schools. Only foolish people think that organized prayer is good for everyone.

TOO PASSIVE I might be wrong, but I think that organized prayer should be discouraged in public schools.

ASSERTIVE TONE Organized prayer should be discouraged in public schools because it violates the religious freedom guaranteed by the First Amendment.

If you are uncertain about the tone of your work, ask for help at your school's writing center.

A2-a Examine your issue's social and intellectual contexts.

Arguments appear in social and intellectual contexts. Public policy debates obviously arise in social contexts. Grounded in specific times and places, such debates are conducted among groups with competing values and interests. For example, the debate over nuclear power plants has been renewed in the United States in light of skyrocketing energy costs and terrorism concerns — with environmentalists, nuclear industry officials, and consumers all weighing in on the argument. Most public policy debates also have intellectual dimensions that address scientific or theoretical questions. In the case of the nuclear power issue, physicists, biologists, and economists all contribute their expertise.

Scholarly debates play out in intellectual contexts, but they have a social dimension too. Scholars and researchers rarely work in a vacuum: They respond to the contributions of other specialists in the field, often building on others' views and refining them, but at times challenging them.

Because many of your readers will be aware of the social and intellectual contexts in which your issue is grounded, you need to conduct some research before preparing your argument; consulting even a few sources can help. For example, the student whose paper appears on pages 74–76 became more knowledgeable about his issue — the ethics of performance-enhancing procedures in sports — after consulting a few brief sources.

A2-b View your audience as a panel of jurors.

Do not assume that your audience already agrees with you; instead, envision skeptical readers who, like a panel of jurors, will make up their minds after listening to all sides of the argument. If you are arguing a public policy issue, aim your paper at readers who represent a variety of opinions. In the case of the debate over nuclear power, for example, imagine a jury representative of those who have a stake in the matter: environmentalists, nuclear industry officials, and consumers.

At times, you can deliberately narrow your audience. If you are working within a word limit, for example, you might not have the space in which to address the concerns of all parties to the nuclear energy debate. Or you might be primarily interested in reaching one segment of a general audience, such as consumers. In such instances, you can still view your audience as a panel of jurors; the jury will simply be a less diverse group.

In the case of scholarly debates, you will be addressing readers who share your interest in a discipline such as literature or psychology. Such readers belong to a group with an agreed-upon way of investigating and talking about issues. Though they generally agree about procedures, scholars in an academic discipline often disagree about particular issues. Once you see how they disagree about your issue, you should be able to imagine a jury that reflects the variety of opinions they hold.

A2-c In your introduction, establish credibility and state your position.

When you construct an argument, make sure your introduction contains a thesis sentence that states your position on the issue you have chosen to debate (see also C2-a). In the sentences leading up to the thesis, establish your credibility with readers by showing that you are knowledgeable and fair-minded. If possible, build common ground with readers who may not be in initial agreement with your views and show them why they need to consider your thesis.

In the following introduction, student Kevin Smith presents himself as someone worth listening to. His opening sentence shows that he is familiar with the legal issues surrounding school prayer. His next sentence reveals him to be fair-minded, as he presents the views of both sides. Even Smith's thesis builds common ground: "Prayer is too important to be trusted to our public schools." Because Smith introduces both sides of the debate, readers are likely to approach his essay with an open mind.

> Although the Supreme Court has ruled against prayer in public schools on First Amendment grounds, many people still feel that prayer should be allowed. Such people value prayer as a practice central to their faith and believe that prayer is a way for schools to reinforce moral principles. They also compellingly point out a paradox in the First Amendment itself: at what point does the separation of church and state restrict the freedom of those who wish to practice their religion? What proponents of school prayer fail to realize, however, is that the Supreme Court's decision, although it was made on legal grounds, makes sense on religious grounds as well. Prayer is too important to be trusted to our public schools.   — Kevin Smith, student

A good way to test a thesis while drafting and revising is to imagine a counterargument to your argument (see A2-f). If you can't think of an opposing point of view, rethink your thesis or ask friends or classmates to respond to your argument.

A2-d Back up your thesis with persuasive lines of argument.

Arguments of any complexity contain lines of argument that, when taken together, might reasonably persuade readers that the thesis has merit. Here, for example, are the main lines of argument used by a student whose thesis was that athletes' use of biotechnology could constitute an unfair advantage in sports.

> Thesis: Athletes who use any type of biotechnology give themselves an unfair advantage and disrupt the sense of fair play, and they should be banned from competition.
>
> - Athletic achievement nowadays increasingly results from biological and high-tech intervention rather than strictly from hard work.
> - There is a difference between the use of state-of-the-art equipment and drugs and the modification of the body itself.
> - If the rules that guarantee an even playing field are violated, competitors and spectators alike are deprived of a sound basis of comparison on which to judge athletic effort and accomplishment.
> - If we let athletes alter their bodies through biotechnology, we might as well dispense with the human element altogether.

If you sum up your main lines of argument, you will have a rough outline of your essay. The outline will consist of your central claim — the thesis — and any supporting claims that back it up. In your paper, you will provide evidence for each of these claims.

ON THE WEB > dianahacker.com/writersref
> Resources for writers and tutors > Tips from writing tutors:
> Writing arguments; Writing essays in English

A2-e Support your claims with specific evidence.

You will need to support your central claim and any subordinate claims with evidence: facts, statistics, examples and illustrations, expert opinion, and so on. Most debatable topics require that you consult some written sources to gather evidence. Always cite your sources. Documentation gives credit to the authors and shows readers how to locate a source in case they want to assess its credibility or explore the issue further (see R4).

Using facts and statistics

A fact is something that is known with certainty because it has been objectively verified: The capital of Wyoming is Cheyenne.

Carbon has an atomic weight of 12. John F. Kennedy was assassinated on November 22, 1963. Statistics are collections of numerical facts: Alcohol abuse is a factor in nearly 40 percent of traffic fatalities. Almost six out of ten US households own a DVD player. As of 2004, about 48 percent of privately held businesses in the United States were owned by women.

Most arguments are supported at least to some extent by facts and statistics. For example, in the following passage the writer uses statistics to show that college students are granted unreasonably high credit limits.

> A 2001 study by Nellie Mae revealed that while the average credit card debt per college undergraduate is $2,327, more than 20% of undergraduates who have at least one credit card maintain a much higher debt level, from $3,000 to $7,000 (Barrett).

Writers and politicians often use statistics in selective ways to bolster their views. If you suspect that a writer's handling of statistics is not quite fair, read authors with opposing views, who may give you a fuller understanding of the numbers.

Using examples and illustrations

Examples and illustrations (extended examples, often in story form) rarely prove a point by themselves, but when used in combination with other forms of evidence they flesh out an argument and bring it to life. Because examples often are vivid, they can reach readers in ways that statistics cannot.

In a paper arguing that any athletes who use gene therapy should be banned from competition, Jamal Hammond gives a thought-provoking example of how running with genetically modified limbs is no different from riding a motorcycle in a footrace.

Citing expert opinion

Although they are no substitute for careful reasoning of your own, the views of an expert can contribute to the force of your argument. For example, to help him make the case that biotechnology could degrade the meaning of sports, Jamal Hammond quotes the remarks of an expert:

> Thomas Murray, chair of the ethics advisory panel for the World Anti-Doping Agency, says he hopes, not too optimistically, for an "alternative future . . . where we still find meaning in great performances as an alchemy of two factors, natural talents . . . and virtues" (qtd. in Jenkins D11).

When you rely on expert opinion, make sure that your source is an authority in the field you are writing about. In some cases you may need to provide credentials showing why your source is worth listening to. When including expert testimony in your paper, you can summarize or paraphrase the expert's opinion or you can quote the expert's exact words. You will of course need to document the source, as in the example just given (see R4).

A2-f Anticipate objections; counter opposing arguments.

Readers who already agree with you need no convincing, although most welcome a well-argued case for their position on an issue. Indifferent or skeptical readers, however, may resist an argument that conflicts with their point of view. In addition to presenting your own case, therefore, you should acknowledge opposing arguments and any contradictory evidence and explain why your position is stronger.

Countering opposing arguments

To anticipate a possible objection, consider the following questions:

- Could a reasonable person draw a different conclusion from your facts or examples?
- Might a reader question any of your assumptions?
- Could a reader offer an alternative explanation of this issue?

To respond to a potential objection, consider these questions:

- Can you concede the point to the opposition but challenge the point's importance or usefulness?
- Can you explain why readers should consider a new perspective or question a piece of evidence?
- Should you qualify your position in light of contradictory evidence?
- Can you suggest a different interpretation of the evidence?

When you write, use phrasing to signal to readers that you're about to present an objection. Often the signal phrase can go in the lead sentence of a paragraph:

- Critics of this view argue that....
- Some readers might point out that....
- Gray presents compelling challenges to....
- But isn't it possible that...?

There is no best place in an essay to deal with opposing views. Often it is useful to summarize the opposing position early in your essay. After stating your thesis but before developing your own arguments, you might have a paragraph that takes up the most important counterargument. Or you can anticipate objections paragraph by paragraph as you develop your case. Wherever you decide to address opposing points of view, explain the arguments of others accurately and fairly.

A2-g Build common ground.

As you counter opposing arguments, try to build common ground with readers who do not initially agree with your views. If you can show that you share your readers' values, they may be able to switch to your position without giving up what they feel is important. For example, to persuade people opposed to shooting deer, a state wildlife commission would have to show that it too cares about preserving deer and does not want them to die needlessly. Having established these values in common, the commission might be able to persuade critics that a carefully controlled hunting season is good for the deer population because it prevents starvation caused by overpopulation.

People believe that intelligence and decency support their side of an argument. To change sides, they must continue to feel intelligent and decent. Otherwise they will persist in their opposition.

A2-h Sample argument paper

In the following paper, student Jamal Hammond argues that we should ban the use of biotechnology by athletes because the practice degrades the values of hard work and natural ability. Notice that he is careful to present opposing views fairly before providing his counterarguments.

In writing the paper, Hammond consulted three newspaper articles, two in print and one online. When he quotes or uses information from a source, he cites the source with an MLA (Modern Language Association) in-text citation. Citations in the paper refer readers to the list of works cited at the end of the paper. (See MLA-4.)

ON THE WEB > dianahacker.com/writersref
Model papers > MLA papers: Orlov; Daly; Levi

Hammond 1

Jamal Hammond

Professor Paschal

English 102

17 March 2006

Performance Enhancement through Biotechnology

Has No Place in Sports

Opening sentences provide background for Hammond's thesis.

The debate over athletes' use of performance-enhancing substances is getting more complicated as biotechnologies such as gene therapy become a reality. The availability of these new methods of boosting performance will force us to decide what we value most in sports--displays of physical excellence developed through hard work or victory at all costs. For centuries, spectators and athletes have cherished the tradition of fairness in sports. While sports competition is, of course, largely about winning, it is also about the means by which a player or team wins.

Thesis states the main point.

Athletes who use any type of biotechnology give themselves an unfair advantage and disrupt the sense of fair play, and they should be banned from competition.

Hammond establishes his credibility by summarizing medical research.

Researchers are experimenting with techniques that could manipulate an athlete's genetic code to build stronger muscles or increase endurance. Searching for cures for diseases like Parkinson's and muscular dystrophy, scientists at the University of Pennsylvania have created "Schwarzenegger mice," rodents that grew larger-than-normal muscles after receiving injections with a gene that stimulates growth protein. The researchers also found that a combination of gene manipulation and exercise led to a 35% increase in the strength of rats'

Source is cited in MLA style.

leg muscles (Lamb 13).

Hammond uses specific evidence to support his thesis.

Such therapies are breakthroughs for humans suffering from muscular diseases; for healthy athletes, they could mean new world records in sports involving speed and endurance--but at what cost to the integrity of athletic competition? The International Olympic Committee's World Anti-Doping Agency has become so alarmed about the possible effects of new gene technology on athletic competition that it has banned the use of gene therapies and urged researchers to devise a test for detecting genetic modification (Lamb 13).

Marginal annotations indicate MLA-style formatting and effective writing.

Hammond 2

Some bioethicists argue that this next wave of performance enhancement is an acceptable and unavoidable feature of competition. As Dr. Andy Miah, who supports the regulated use of gene therapies in sports, claims, "The idea of the naturally perfect athlete is romantic nonsense. . . . An athlete achieves what he or she achieves through all sorts of means-- technology, sponsorship, support and so on" (qtd. in Rudebeck). Miah, in fact, sees athletes' imminent turn to genetic modification as "merely a continuation of the way sport works; it allows us to create more extraordinary performances" (Rudebeck). Miah's approval of "extraordinary performances" as the goal of competition reflects our culture's tendency to demand and reward new heights of athletic achievement. The problem is that achievement nowadays increasingly results from biological and high-tech intervention rather than strictly from hard work.

Better equipment, such as aerodynamic bicycles and fiberglass poles for pole vaulting, have made it possible for athletes to record achievements unthinkable a generation ago. But athletes themselves must put forth the physical effort of training and practice--they must still build their skills--even in the murky area of legal and illegal drug use (Jenkins D11). There is a difference between the use of state-of-the-art equipment and drugs and the modification of the body itself. Athletes who use medical technology to alter their bodies can bypass the hard work of training by taking on the powers of a machine. If they set new records this way, we lose the opportunity to witness sports as a spectacle of human effort and are left marveling at scientific advances, which have little relation to the athletic tradition of fair play.

Such a tradition has long defined athletic competition. Sports rely on equal conditions to ensure fair play, from regulations that demand similar equipment to referees who evenhandedly apply the rules to all participants. If the rules that guarantee an even playing field are violated, competitors and spectators alike are deprived of a sound basis of comparison on which to judge athletic effort and accomplishment. When major league baseball rules call for solid-wood bats, the player who uses a corked bat enhances his hitting statistics at the expense of players who use regulation equipment. When Ben Johnson tested

Opposing views are presented fairly.

"Qtd. in" is used for an indirect source: words quoted in another source.

Hammond counters opposing arguments.

Hammond develops the thesis.

Transition moves from the writer's main argument to specific examples.

Hammond 3

positive for steroids after setting a world record in the 100-meter dash in
the 1988 Olympics, his "achievement" devalued the intense training that
his competitors had undergone to prepare for the event--and the International Olympic Committee responded by stripping Johnson of his medal
and his world record. Likewise, athletes who use gene therapy to alter their
bodies and enhance their performance will create an uneven playing field.

A vivid example
helps the writer
make his point.

If we let athletes alter their bodies through biotechnology, we might
as well dispense with the human element altogether. Instead of watching
the 100-meter dash to see who the fastest runner in the world is, we might
just as well watch the sprinters mount motorcycles and race across the
finish line. The absurdity of such an example, however, points to the
damage that we will do to sports if we allow these therapies. Thomas
Murray, chair of the ethics advisory panel for the World Anti-Doping
Agency, says he hopes, not too optimistically, for an "alternative future . . .
where we still find meaning in great performances as an alchemy of two
factors, natural talents . . . and virtues" (qtd. in Jenkins D11).

Conclusion echoes
the thesis without
dully repeating it.

Unless we are willing to organize separate sporting events and
leagues--an Olympics, say, for athletes who have opted for a boost from the
test tube and another for athletes who have chosen to keep their bodies
natural--we should ask from our athletes that they dazzle us less with
extraordinary performance and more with the fruits of their hard work.

Hammond 4

Works Cited

Works cited page
uses MLA style.

Jenkins, Sally. "The First Item in a Pandora's Box of Moral
    Ambiguities." Washington Post 4 Dec. 2004: D11.
Lamb, Gregory M. "Will Gene-Altered Athletes Kill Sports?" Christian
    Science Monitor 23 Aug. 2004: 12-13.
Rudebeck, Clare. "The Eyes Have It." Independent [London] 27 Apr.
    2005. 28 Feb. 2006 <http://news.independent.co.uk/world/
    science_technology/article3597.ece>.

A3

Evaluating arguments

In your reading and in your own writing, evaluate all arguments for logic and fairness. Many arguments can stand up to critical scrutiny. Often, however, a line of argument that at first seems reasonable turns out to be fallacious, unfair, or both.

ON THE WEB > dianahacker.com/writersref
Additional resources > Links Library > Argument

A3-a Distinguish between reasonable and fallacious argumentative tactics.

A number of unreasonable argumentative tactics are known as *logical fallacies*. Most of the fallacies — such as hasty generalizations and false analogies — are misguided or dishonest uses of legitimate argumentative strategies. The examples in this section suggest when such strategies are reasonable and when they are not.

Generalizing (inductive reasoning)

Writers and thinkers generalize all the time. We look at a sample of data and conclude that data we have not observed will most likely conform to what we have seen before. From a spoonful of soup, we conclude just how salty the whole bowl will be. After numerous bad experiences with an airline, we decide to book future flights with one of its competitors instead.

When we draw a conclusion from an array of facts, we are engaged in inductive reasoning. Such reasoning deals in probability, not certainty. For a conclusion to be highly probable, it must be based on evidence that is sufficient, representative, and relevant. (See the chart on p. 79.)

The fallacy known as *hasty generalization* is a conclusion based on insufficient or unrepresentative evidence.

HASTY GENERALIZATION

Deaths from drug overdoses in Metropolis have doubled in the past three years. Therefore, more Americans than ever are dying from drug abuse.

Data from one city do not justify a conclusion about the whole United States.

A *stereotype* is a hasty generalization about a group. Here are a few examples.

STEREOTYPES

Women are bad bosses.

Politicians are corrupt.

Asian students are exceptionally intelligent.

Stereotyping is common because of our human tendency to perceive selectively. We tend to see what we want to see; that is, we notice evidence confirming our already formed opinions and fail to notice evidence to the contrary. For example, if you have concluded that politicians are corrupt, your stereotype will be confirmed by news reports of legislators being indicted — even though every day the media describe conscientious officials serving the public honestly and well.

NOTE: Many hasty generalizations contain words like *all, ever, always,* and *never,* when qualifiers such as *most, many, usually,* and *seldom* would be more accurate.

Drawing analogies

An analogy points out a similarity between two things that are otherwise different. Analogies can be an effective means of arguing a point. In fact, our system of case law, which relies heavily on precedents, makes extensive use of reasoning by analogy. A prosecutor may argue, for example, that Z is guilty because his actions resemble those of X and Y, who were judged guilty in previous rulings. In response, the defense may maintain that the actions of Z bear only a superficial resemblance to those of X and Y and that in legally relevant respects they are in fact quite different.

It is not always easy to draw the line between a reasonable and an unreasonable analogy. At times, however, an analogy is clearly off-base, in which case it is called a *false analogy.*

FALSE ANALOGY

If we can put humans on the moon, we should be able to find a cure for the common cold.

The writer has falsely assumed that because two things are alike in one respect, they must be alike in others. Putting human beings on the moon and finding a cure for the common cold are both scientific

Testing inductive reasoning

Though inductive reasoning leads to probable and not absolute truth, you can assess a conclusion's likely probability by asking three questions. This chart shows how to apply those questions to a sample conclusion based on a survey.

CONCLUSION   The majority of students on our campus would subscribe to wireless Internet access if it were available.

EVIDENCE   In a recent survey, 923 of 1,515 students questioned say they would subscribe to wireless Internet access.

1. Is the evidence sufficient?
   That depends. On a small campus (say, 3,000 students), the pool of students surveyed would be sufficient for market research, but on a large campus (say, 30,000), 1,515 students are only 5 percent of the population. If that 5 percent were known to be truly representative of the other 95 percent, however, even such a small sample would be sufficient (see question 2).

2. Is the evidence representative?
   The evidence is representative if those responding to the survey reflect the characteristics of the entire student population: age, sex, level of technical expertise, amount of disposable income, and so on. If most of those surveyed are majoring in technical fields, for example, the researchers would be wise to question the survey's conclusion.

3. Is the evidence relevant?
   The answer is yes. The results of the survey are directly linked to the conclusion. A question about the number of hours spent on the Internet, by contrast, would not be relevant, because it would not be about *subscribing to wireless Internet access.*

challenges, but the technical problems confronting medical researchers are quite different from those solved by space scientists.

Tracing causes and effects

Demonstrating a connection between causes and effects is rarely a simple matter. For example, to explain why a chemistry course has a high failure rate, you would begin by listing possible causes: inadequate preparation of students, poor teaching, large class size, lack of qualified tutors, and so on. Next you would investigate each possible cause. To see whether inadequate preparation contributes to the high failure rate, for instance, you might compare the math and science backgrounds of successful and failing students. To see whether large class size is a contributing factor, you might run a pilot program of small classes and compare grades in the small classes with those in the larger ones. Only after investigating the possible causes would you be able to weigh the relative impact of each cause and suggest appropriate remedies.

Because cause-and-effect reasoning is so complex, it is not surprising that writers frequently oversimplify it. In particular, writers sometimes assume that because one event follows another, the first is the cause of the second. This common fallacy is known as *post hoc*, from the Latin *post hoc, ergo propter hoc*, meaning "after this, therefore because of this."

POST HOC FALLACY

Since Governor Cho took office, unemployment of minorities in the state has decreased by 7 percent. Governor Cho should be applauded for reducing unemployment among minorities.

The writer must show that Governor Cho's policies are responsible for the decrease in unemployment; it is not enough to show that the decrease followed the governor's taking office.

Weighing options

Especially when reasoning about problems and solutions, writers must weigh options. To be fair, a writer should mention the full range of options, showing why one is superior to the others or might work well in combination with others.

It is unfair to suggest that there are only two alternatives when in fact there are more. Writers who set up a false choice between their preferred option and one that is clearly unsatisfactory are guilty of the *either . . . or* fallacy.

EITHER . . . OR FALLACY

Our current war against drugs has not worked. Either we should legalize drugs or we should turn the drug war over to our armed forces and let them fight it.

Clearly there are other options, such as increased funding for drug prevention and treatment.

Making assumptions

An assumption is a claim that is taken to be true — without the need of proof. Most arguments are based to some extent on assumptions, since writers rarely have the time and space to prove all of the conceivable claims on which an argument is based. For example, someone arguing about the best means of limiting population growth in developing countries might well assume that the goal of limiting population growth is worthwhile. For most audiences, there would be no need to articulate this assumption or to defend it.

There is a danger, however, in failing to spell out and prove a claim that is clearly controversial. Consider the following short argument, in which a key claim is missing.

ARGUMENT WITH MISSING CLAIM

Violent crime is increasing.

Therefore, we should vigorously enforce the death penalty.

The writer seems to be assuming that the death penalty deters violent criminals — and that most audiences will agree. Obviously, neither is a safe assumption.

When a missing claim is an assertion that few would agree with, we say that a writer is guilty of a *non sequitur* (Latin for "does not follow").

NON SEQUITUR

Mary loves good food; therefore, she will be an excellent chef.

Few people would agree with the missing claim — that lovers of good food always make excellent chefs.

Deducing conclusions (deductive reasoning)

When we deduce a conclusion, we — like Sherlock Holmes — put things together. We establish that a general principle is true, that a specific case is an example of that principle, and that therefore a particular conclusion is a certainty. In real life, such absolute reasoning rarely happens. Approximations of it, however, sometimes occur.

Deductive reasoning can often be structured in a three-step argument called a *syllogism*. The three steps are the major premise, the minor premise, and the conclusion.

1. Anything that increases radiation in the environment is dangerous to public health. (Major premise)
2. Nuclear reactors increase radiation in the environment. (Minor premise)
3. Therefore, nuclear reactors are dangerous to public health. (Conclusion)

The major premise is a generalization. The minor premise is a specific case. The conclusion follows from applying the generalization to the specific case.

Deductive arguments break down if one of the premises is not true or if the conclusion does not logically follow from the premises. In the following short argument, the major premise is very likely untrue.

ARGUMENT WITH A QUESTIONABLE PREMISE

The police do not give speeding tickets to people driving less than five miles per hour over the limit. Sam is driving fifty-nine miles per hour in a fifty-five-mile-per-hour zone. Therefore, the police will not give Sam a speeding ticket.

The conclusion is true only if the premises are true. If the police sometimes give tickets for less than five-mile-per-hour violations, Sam cannot safely conclude that he will avoid a ticket.

In the following argument, both premises might be true, but the conclusion does not follow logically from them.

CONCLUSION DOES NOT FOLLOW

All members of our club ran in this year's Boston Marathon. Jay ran in this year's Boston Marathon. Therefore, Jay is a member of our club.

The fact that Jay ran the marathon is no guarantee that he is a member of the club. Presumably, many runners are nonmembers.

Assuming that both premises are true, the following argument holds up.

CONCLUSION FOLLOWS

All members of our club ran in this year's Boston Marathon. Jay is a member of our club. Therefore, Jay ran in this year's Boston Marathon.

A3-b Distinguish between legitimate and unfair emotional appeals.

There is nothing wrong with appealing to readers' emotions. After all, many issues worth arguing about have an emotional as well as a logical dimension. Even the Greek logician Aristotle lists *pathos* (emotion) as a legitimate argumentative tactic. For example, in an essay criticizing big-box stores, writer Betsy Taylor has a good reason for tugging at readers' emotions: Her subject is the decline of city and town life. In her conclusion, Taylor appeals to readers' emotions by invoking their national pride.

LEGITIMATE EMOTIONAL APPEAL

Is it anti-American to be against having a retail giant set up shop in one's community? Some people would say so. On the other hand, if you board up Main Street, what's left of America?

As we all know, however, emotional appeals are frequently misused. Many of the arguments we see in the media, for instance, strive to win our sympathy rather than our intelligent agreement. A TV commercial suggesting that you will be thin and sexy if you drink a certain diet beverage is making a pitch to emotions. So is a political speech that recommends electing a candidate because he is a devoted husband and father who serves as a volunteer firefighter. The following passage illustrates several types of unfair emotional appeals.

UNFAIR EMOTIONAL APPEALS

This progressive proposal to build a ski resort in the state park has been carefully researched by Western Trust, the largest bank in the state; furthermore, it is favored by a majority of the local merchants. The only opposition comes from narrow-minded, do-gooder environmentalists who care more about trees than they do about people; one of their leaders was actually arrested for disturbing the peace several years ago.

Words with strong positive or negative connotations, such as *progressive* and *do-gooder*, are examples of *biased language*. Attacking the persons who hold a belief (environmentalists) rather than refuting their argument is called *ad hominem*, a Latin term meaning "to the man." Associating a prestigious name (Western Trust) with the writer's side is called *transfer*. Claiming that an idea should be accepted because a large number of people are in favor (the majority of merchants) is called the *bandwagon appeal*. Bringing in irrelevant issues (the arrest) is a *red herring*, named after a trick used in fox hunts to mislead the dogs by dragging a smelly fish across the trail.

A3-c Judge how fairly a writer handles opposing views.

The way in which a writer deals with opposing views is telling. Some writers address the arguments of the opposition fairly, conceding points when necessary and countering others, all in a civil spirit. Other writers will do almost anything to win an argument: either ignoring opposing views altogether or misrepresenting such views and attacking their proponents.

In your own writing, you build credibility by addressing opposing arguments fairly. (See also A2-f.) In your reading, you can assess the credibility of your sources by looking at how they deal with views not in agreement with their own.

Describing the views of others

Writers and politicians often deliberately misrepresent the views of others. One way they do this is by setting up a "straw man," a character so weak that he is easily knocked down. The *straw man* fallacy consists of an oversimplification or outright distortion of opposing views. For example, in a California debate over attempts to control the mountain lion population, pro-lion groups characterized their opponents as trophy hunters bent on shooting harmless lions and sticking them on the walls of their dens. In truth, such hunters were only one faction of those who saw a need to control the lion population.

In response to the District of Columbia's request for voting representation, some politicians have set up a straw man, as shown in the following example.

STRAW MAN FALLACY

Washington, DC, residents are lobbying for statehood. Giving a city such as the District of Columbia the status of a state would be unfair.

The straw man wants statehood. In fact, most District citizens are lobbying for voting representation in any form, not necessarily through statehood.

Quoting opposing views

Writers often quote the words of writers who hold opposing views. In general, this is a good idea, for it assures some level of fairness and accuracy. At times, though, both the fairness and accuracy are an illusion.

A source may be misrepresented when it is quoted out of context. All quotations are to some extent taken out of context, but a fair writer will explain the context to readers. To select a provocative sentence from a source and to ignore the more moderate sentences surrounding it is both unfair and misleading. Sometimes a writer deliberately distorts a source through the device of ellipsis dots. Ellipsis dots tell readers that words have been omitted from the original source (see P7-g). When those words are crucial to an author's meaning, omitting them is obviously unfair.

ORIGINAL SOURCE

Johnson's *History of the American West* is riddled with inaccuracies and astonishing in its blatantly racist description of the Indian wars.   — B. Smith, reviewer

MISLEADING QUOTATION

According to B. Smith, Johnson's *History of the American West* is "astonishing in its . . . description of the Indian wars."

A4

Writing in the disciplines

College courses expose you to the thinking of scholars in many disciplines, such as the humanities (literature, music, art), the social sciences (psychology, anthropology, sociology), and the sciences (biology, physics, chemistry). Writing in any discipline provides the opportunity to practice the methods used by scholars in these fields and to enter into their debates. Each field has its own questions, evidence, language, and conventions, but all disciplines share certain expectations for good writing.

A4-a   Find commonalities across disciplines.

A good paper in any field needs to communicate a writer's purpose to an audience and to explore an engaging question about a subject (see C1-a). All effective writers make an argument and support their claims with evidence (see A2-e). Writers in any field need to show readers the thesis they're developing (or, in the sciences, the hypothesis they're testing) and how they counter opposing explanations or objections of other writers (see A2-f). All disciplines require writers to document where they found their evidence and from whom they borrowed ideas (see A4-e).

A4-b   Recognize the questions writers in a discipline ask.

Disciplines are characterized by the kinds of questions their scholars attempt to answer. One way to understand how disciplines ask different questions is to look at assignments on the same topic in various fields. Many disciplines, for example, might be interested in cults. The questions on the next page show how writers in different fields approach the topic of cults.

SOCIOLOGY	What role does gender play in cult leadership?
HISTORY	Why did the cult of Caesar take hold in ancient Rome?
FILM	How does the movie *Fight Club* portray contemporary cults?
BIOLOGY	Do individuals susceptible to cult influence share genetic characteristics?
BUSINESS	How do multilevel marketing (MLM) practices depend on cult techniques for their success?

The questions you will ask in any discipline will form the basis of the thesis for your paper. Questions themselves don't communicate a central idea, but they may lead you to one. For example, the historian who asks "Why did the cult of Caesar take hold in ancient Rome?" might work out a thesis like this: *By raising Caesar to the status of a deity, imperial Rome attempted to unify the various peoples in its far-flung realm into one cult of worship centered on the emperor.*

A4-c Understand the kinds of evidence writers in a discipline use.

Regardless of the discipline in which you're writing, you must support any claims you make with evidence — facts, statistics, examples and illustrations, expert opinion, and so on.

The kinds of evidence used in different disciplines commonly overlap. Students of geography, media studies, and political science, for example, all might use census data to explore different topics. The evidence that one discipline values, however, might not be sufficient to support an interpretation or a conclusion in another field. For example, psychologists, who look for evidence in case studies and in the results of experiments, seldom use expert opinion as evidence. The chart at the top of the next page lists the kinds of evidence typically used in various disciplines.

A4-d Become familiar with a discipline's language conventions.

Every discipline has a specialized vocabulary. As you read the articles and books in a field, you'll notice certain words and phrases that come up repeatedly. Sociologists, for example, use terms like

Evidence typically used in various disciplines

Humanities: Literature, art, film, music, philosophy
- Passages of text or lines of a poem
- Details from an image or a work of art
- Passages of a musical composition
- Essays that analyze original works or put forth theories

Humanities: History
- Firsthand sources such as photographs, letters, maps, and government documents
- Scholarly books and articles that interpret evidence

Social sciences: Psychology, sociology, political science, anthropology
- Data from original experiments
- Results of field research such as interviews, observations, or surveys
- Statistics from government agencies
- Scholarly books and articles that interpret data from original experiments and from other researchers' studies

Sciences: Biology, chemistry, physics
- Data from original experiments
- Scholarly articles that report findings from experiments

independent variables, political opportunity resources, and *dyads* to describe social phenomena; computer scientists might refer to *algorithm design* and *loop invariants* to describe programming methods. Practitioners in health fields such as nursing use terms like *treatment plan* and *systemic assessment* to describe patient care. Use discipline-specific terms only when you are certain that you and your readers fully understand their meaning.

In addition to vocabulary, many fields of study have developed specialized conventions for point of view and verb tense. See the chart on the next page.

A4-e Use a discipline's preferred citation style.

In any discipline, you must give credit to those whose ideas or words you have borrowed. Avoid plagiarism by citing sources honestly and accurately (see R4).

Point of view and verb tense in academic writing

Point of view

- Writers of analytical or research essays in the humanities usually use the third-person point of view: *Austen presents . . .* or *Castel describes the battle as. . . .*

- Scientists and most social scientists, who depend on quantitative research to present findings, tend to use the third-person point of view: *The results indicated. . . .*

- Writers in the humanities and in some social sciences occasionally use the first person in discussing their personal experience or in writing a personal narrative: *After spending two years interviewing families affected by the war, I began to understand that . . .* or *Every July as we approached the Cape Cod Canal, we could sense. . . .*

Present or past tense

- Literature scholars use the present tense to discuss a text: *Hughes effectively dramatizes different views of minority assertiveness.* (See MLA-3.)

- Science and social science writers use the past tense to describe experiments and the present tense to discuss the findings: *In 2003, Berkowitz released the first double-blind placebo study. . . . These results paint a murky picture.* (See APA-3.)

- Writers in history use the present tense or the present perfect tense to discuss a text: *Shelby Foote describes the scene like this . . .* or *Shelby Foote has described the scene like this. . . .* (See CMS-3.)

While all disciplines emphasize careful documentation, each follows a particular system of citation that its members have agreed on. Writers in the humanities usually use the system established by the Modern Language Association (MLA). Scholars in some social sciences, such as psychology and anthropology, follow the style guidelines of the American Psychological Association (APA); scholars in history and some humanities typically follow *The Chicago Manual of Style*. For guidance on using the MLA, APA, or *Chicago* (CMS) format, see MLA-4, APA-4, or CMS-4, respectively.

Approaching assignments in the disciplines

When you receive a writing assignment, look for key terms that alert you to the purpose of the assignment and to the specialized language of the field. Also determine the kinds of evidence that would be appropriate to support your argument. At first glance, the following four assignments might seem to have nothing in common. A closer look will show that they all use key terms specific to the field, they all use the vocabulary of the field to describe the purpose of the assignment, and they all explain or suggest the kinds of evidence the writers should use.

Environmental science

The El Niño Southern Oscillation (ENSO) is a worldwide climatic oscillation. Evaluate the scientific issues involved in enhancing our ability to predict ENSO events and current limitations to our forecasting ability. Use scientific papers, abstracts, review articles, and course readings to support your conclusions.

1. Key terms
2. Purpose: to summarize and analyze research findings
3. Appropriate evidence: articles, visuals, especially conflicting data

Business

Develop a position in response to the following question: Do corporate takeovers create or destroy value? To determine how these value changes come about, analyze case studies and Securities and Exchange Commission documents.

1. Key terms
2. Purpose: to analyze certain evidence and to argue a position based on that analysis
3. Appropriate evidence: examples of corporate takeovers

Approaching assignments in the disciplines (continued)

Anthropology

┌────────2────────┐   ┌──────1──────┐
Compare and contrast the male rites of passage among the Sambia of

                                                  ┌────1────┐
New Guinea and the Maasai of southern Kenya. Consult ethnographic

┌──────────────────────3──────────────────────┐
descriptions of Sambian and Maasai rituals in course readings.

1. Key terms
2. Purpose: to analyze similarities and differences
3. Appropriate evidence: anthropologists' field research

Nursing

┌──2──┐   ┌────1────┐
Compile a detailed, objective health history for a member of your

            ┌──────────────3──────────────┐
family. Use interview notes and any available health records to build

the patient history.

1. Key term
2. Purpose: to record information
3. Appropriate evidence: interviews, relevant health records

    Once you have determined the expectations of a writing assignment, you must be sure to do the following, regardless of the discipline you are writing in.

- Determine your audience and purpose (see C1-a).
- Ask questions appropriate to the field (see A4-b).
- Formulate a thesis (see C2-a).
- Gather evidence. Conduct research if necessary (see R1).
- Identify the required citation style (see R4).

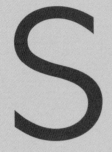

S

Sentence Style

S Sentence Style

S1

Parallelism

If two or more ideas are parallel, they are easier to grasp when expressed in parallel grammatical form. Single words should be balanced with single words, phrases with phrases, clauses with clauses.

> A kiss can be a comma, a question mark, or an exclamation point.
> —Mistinguett

> This novel is not to be tossed lightly aside, but to be hurled with great force.
> —Dorothy Parker

> In matters of principle, stand like a rock; in matters of taste, swim with the current.
> —Thomas Jefferson

GRAMMAR CHECKERS only occasionally flag faulty parallelism. Because the programs cannot assess whether ideas are parallel in grammatical form, they fail to catch the faulty parallelism in sentences such as this: *In my high school, boys were either jocks, preppies, or studied constantly.*

S1-a Balance parallel ideas in a series.

Readers expect items in a series to appear in parallel grammatical form. When one or more of the items violate readers' expectations, a sentence will be needlessly awkward.

▶ Abused children commonly exhibit one or more of the following symptoms: withdrawal, rebelliousness, restlessness, and
depression.
~~they are depressed.~~
  ^

The revision presents all of the items as nouns.

▶ Hooked on romance novels, I learned that nothing is more
  having
  important than being rich, looking good, and ~~to have~~ a good
  ^
  time.

The revision uses *-ing* forms for all items in the series.

▶ After assuring us that he was sober, Sam drove down the middle
  went through
  of the road, ran one red light, and two stop signs.
  ^

The revision adds a verb to make the three items parallel: *drove...,*
ran ..., went through. ...

NOTE: For parallelism in headings and lists, see C5-b and C5-c.

S1-b Balance parallel ideas presented as pairs.

When pairing ideas, underscore their connection by expressing
them in similar grammatical form. Paired ideas are usually connected in one of these ways:

- with a coordinating conjunction such as *and, but,* or *or*
- with a pair of correlative conjunctions such as *either...or*
  or *not only...but also*
- with a word introducing a comparison, usually *than* or *as*

Parallel ideas linked with coordinating conjunctions

Coordinating conjunctions (*and, but, or, nor, for, so,* and *yet*) link
ideas of equal importance. When those ideas are closely parallel in
content, they should be expressed in parallel grammatical form.

▶ At Lincoln High School, vandalism can result in suspension
  expulsion
  or even ~~being expelled~~ from school.
  ^

The revision balances the nouns *suspension* and *expulsion.*

▶ Many states are reducing property taxes for home owners and
  extending
  ~~extend~~ financial aid in the form of tax credits to renters.
  ^

The revision balances the *-ing* verb forms *reducing* and *extending.*

Parallel ideas linked with correlative conjunctions

Correlative conjunctions come in pairs: *either. . . or, neither. . . nor, not only. . . but also, both . . . and, whether. . . or.* Make sure that the grammatical structure following the second half of the pair is the same as that following the first half.

▶ Thomas Edison was not only a prolific inventor but also ~~was~~ a

successful entrepreneur.

A prolific inventor follows *not only,* so *a successful entrepreneur* should follow *but also.* Repeating *was* creates an unbalanced effect.

▶ The clerk told me either to change my flight or ^{to} take the train.

To change my flight, which follows *either,* should be balanced with *to take the train,* which follows *or.*

Comparisons linked with than *or* as

In comparisons linked with *than* or *as,* the elements being compared should be expressed in parallel grammatical structure.

▶ It is easier to speak in abstractions than ^{to ground} ~~grounding~~ one's thoughts

in reality.

▶ Mother could not persuade me that giving is as much a joy as
receiving.
~~to receive.~~

To speak in abstractions is balanced with *to ground one's thoughts in reality. Giving* is balanced with *receiving.*

NOTE: Comparisons should also be logical and complete. See S2-c.

S1-c Repeat function words to clarify parallels.

Function words such as prepositions (*by, to*) and subordinating conjunctions (*that, because*) signal the grammatical nature of the word groups to follow. Although they can sometimes be omitted, include them whenever they signal parallel structures that might otherwise be missed by readers.

▶ Many hooked smokers try switching to a brand they find
   to
distasteful or a low tar and nicotine cigarette.
            ^

In the original sentence, the prepositional phrase was too complex for easy reading. The repetition of the preposition *to* prevents readers from losing their way.

ON THE WEB > dianahacker.com/writersref
Grammar exercises > Sentence style > E-ex S1–1 through S1–3

S2

Needed words

Do not omit words necessary for grammatical or logical completeness. Readers need to see at a glance how the parts of a sentence are connected.

> **ESL**   Languages sometimes differ in the need for certain words. In particular, be alert for missing articles, verbs, subjects, or expletives. See E3, E2-a, and E2-b.

> ✔   GRAMMAR CHECKERS do not flag the vast majority of missing words. They can, however, catch some missing verbs (see G2-e). Although they can flag some missing articles (*a, an,* and *the*), they often suggest that an article is missing when in fact it is not. (See also E3.)

S2-a   Add words needed to complete compound structures.

In compound structures, words are often omitted for economy: *Tom is a man who means what he says and [who] says what he means.* Such omissions are perfectly acceptable as long as the omitted word is common to both parts of the compound structure.

If the shorter version defies grammar or idiom because an omitted word is not common to both parts of the compound structure, the word must be put back in.

▶ Some of the regulars are acquaintances whom we see at work or
who
^
live in our community.

The word *who* must be included because *whom . . . live in our commu-nity* is not grammatically correct.

accepted
▶ Mayor Davis never has and never will accept a bribe from
^
anyone.

Has . . . accept is not grammatically correct.

in
▶ Many South Pacific tribes still believe and live by ancient laws.
^
Believe . . . by is not idiomatic English.

S2-b Add the word *that* if there is any danger of misreading without it.

If there is no danger of misreading, the word *that* may sometimes be omitted when it introduces a subordinate clause: *The value of a principle is the number of things [that] it will explain.* Occasionally, however, a sentence might be misread without *that.*

that
▶ Looking out the family room window, Sarah saw her favorite tree,
^
which she had climbed so often as a child, was gone.

Sarah didn't see the tree; she saw that the tree was gone. The word *that* tells readers to expect a clause, not just *tree,* as the direct object of *saw.*

S2-c Add words needed to make comparisons logical and complete.

Comparisons should be made between items that are alike. To com-pare unlike items is illogical and distracting.

▶ The forests of North America are much more extensive than
those of
Europe.
^
Forests must be compared with forests.

▶ *Our*   *graduate at a higher rate*
~~The graduation rate of our~~ student athletes ~~is higher~~ than the
rest of the student population.

A rate cannot be logically compared with a population. The writer could revise the sentence by inserting *that of* after *than,* but the preceding revision is more concise.

▶ Some say that Ella Fitzgerald's renditions of Cole Porter's songs
singer's.
are better than any other ~~singer.~~

Ella Fitzgerald's renditions cannot be logically compared with a singer. The revision uses the possessive form *singer's,* with the word *renditions* being implied.

Sometimes the word *other* must be inserted to make a comparison logical.

other
▶ Jupiter is larger than any planet in our solar system.

Jupiter cannot be larger than itself.

Sometimes the word *as* must be inserted to make a comparison grammatically correct.

as
▶ The city of Lowell is as old, if not older than, the city of Lawrence.

The construction *as old* is not complete without a second *as: as old as . . . the city of Lawrence.*

Comparisons should be complete enough so that readers will understand what is being compared.

INCOMPLETE   Brand X is less salty.

COMPLETE   Brand X is less salty than Brand Y.

Also, comparisons should leave no ambiguity for readers. If more than one interpretation is possible, revise the sentence to state clearly which interpretation you intend. In the following sentence, two interpretations are possible.

AMBIGUOUS   Ken helped me more than my roommate.

CLEAR   Ken helped me more than *he helped* my roommate.

CLEAR   Ken helped me more than my roommate *did.*

S2-d Add the articles *a, an,* and *the* where necessary for grammatical completeness.

Articles are sometimes omitted in recipes and other instructions that are meant to be followed while they are being read. Such omissions are inappropriate, however, in nearly all other forms of writing, whether formal or informal.

> ▶ Blood can be drawn only by doctor or by authorized person
> who has been trained in procedure.

(with handwritten insertions: a, an, the)

It is not always necessary to repeat articles with paired items: *We bought a computer and printer.* However, if one of the items requires *a* and the other requires *an,* both articles must be included.

> ▶ We bought a computer and antivirus program at a
> discount.

(with handwritten insertion: an)

ON THE WEB > dianahacker.com/writersref
Grammar exercises > Sentence style > E-ex S2–1 and S2–2

S3

Problems with modifiers

Modifiers, whether they are single words, phrases, or clauses, should point clearly to the words they modify. As a rule, related words should be kept together.

> ✓ GRAMMAR CHECKERS can flag split infinitives, such as *to carefully and thoroughly sift* (S3-d). However, they don't alert you to other misplaced modifiers (*I only ate three radishes*) or dangling modifiers, including danglers like this one: *When a young man, my mother enrolled me in tap dance classes, hoping I would become the next Savion Glover.*

S3-a Put limiting modifiers in front of the words they modify.

Limiting modifiers such as *only, even, almost, nearly,* and *just* should appear in front of a verb only if they modify the verb: *At first I couldn't even touch my toes, much less grasp them.* If they limit the meaning of some other word in the sentence, they should be placed in front of that word.

> Lasers ~~only~~ destroy$\overset{\textit{only}}{\wedge}$ the target, leaving the surrounding healthy tissue intact.

Only limits the meaning of *the target,* not *destroy.*

> The turtle ~~only~~ makes progress$\overset{\textit{only}}{\wedge}$ when it sticks its neck out.

Only limits the meaning of the *when* clause.

When the limiting modifier *not* is misplaced, the sentence usually suggests a meaning the writer did not intend.

> In the United States in 1860, all black southerners were$\overset{\textit{not}}{\wedge}$ ~~not~~ slaves.

The original sentence says that no black southerners were slaves. The revision makes the writer's real meaning clear: Some (but not all) black southerners were slaves.

S3-b Place phrases and clauses so that readers can see at a glance what they modify.

Although phrases and clauses can appear at some distance from the words they modify, make sure that your meaning is clear. When phrases or clauses are oddly placed, absurd misreadings can result.

MISPLACED   The soccer player returned to the clinic where he had undergone emergency surgery in 2004 in a limousine sent by Adidas.

REVISED   Traveling in a limousine sent by Adidas, the soccer player returned to the clinic where he had undergone emergency surgery in 2004.

The revision corrects the false impression that the soccer player underwent emergency surgery in a limousine.

▶ *On the walls*
~~There~~ are many pictures of comedians who have performed at
  ^

Gavin's. ~~on the walls.~~
              ^

The comedians weren't performing on the walls; the pictures were on the walls.

▶ The robber was described as a six-foot-tall *150-pound,* man with a mustache.
                                    ^   ^
~~weighing 150 pounds.~~

The robber, not the mustache, weighed 150 pounds.

Occasionally the placement of a modifier leads to an ambiguity, in which case two revisions will be possible, depending on the writer's intended meaning.

AMBIGUOUS   The exchange students we met for coffee occasionally questioned us about our latest slang.

CLEAR   The exchange students we occasionally met for coffee questioned us about our latest slang.

CLEAR   The exchange students we met for coffee questioned us occasionally about our latest slang.

In the original version, it was not clear whether the meeting or the questioning happened occasionally. The revisions eliminate the ambiguity.

S3-c Move awkwardly placed modifiers.

As a rule, a sentence should flow from subject to verb to object, without lengthy detours along the way. When a long adverbial element separates a subject from its verb, a verb from its object, or a helping verb from its main verb, the result is often awkward.

▶ *A*
~~Hong Kong,~~ after more than 150 years of British rule, was *Hong Kong*
                ^   ^

transferred back to Chinese control in 1997.

There is no reason to separate the subject, *Hong Kong,* from the verb, *was transferred,* with a long adverb phrase.

EXCEPTION: Occasionally a writer may choose to delay a verb or an object to create suspense. In the following passage, for example, Robert Mueller inserts the *after* phrase between the subject, *women,* and the verb, *walk,* to heighten the dramatic effect.

> I asked a Burmese why women, after centuries of following their men, now walk ahead. He said there were many unexploded land mines since the war.   —Robert Mueller

---

ESL   English does not allow an adverb to appear between a verb and its object. See E2-f.

        easily
▶ Yolanda lifted ~~easily~~ the fifty-pound weight.
        ^

S3-d Avoid split infinitives when they are awkward.

An infinitive consists of *to* plus a verb: *to think, to breathe, to dance.* When a modifier appears between its two parts, an infinitive is said to be "split": *to carefully balance, to completely understand.*

When a long word or a phrase appears between the parts of the infinitive, the result is usually awkward.

    If possible, patients
▶ ~~Patients~~ should try to ~~if possible~~ avoid going up and down stairs
   ^

by themselves.

Attempts to avoid split infinitives can result in equally awkward sentences. When alternative phrasing sounds unnatural, most experts allow—and even encourage—splitting the infinitive.

    AWKWARD   We decided actually to enforce the law.

    BETTER   We decided to actually enforce the law.

At times, neither the split infinitive nor its alternative sounds particularly awkward. In such situations, you may want to unsplit the infinitive, especially in formal writing.

                                        formally.
▶ The candidate decided to ~~formally~~ launch her campaign/
                                           ^

ON THE WEB > dianahacker.com/writersref
    Language Debates > Split infinitives

S3-e Repair dangling modifiers.

A dangling modifier fails to refer logically to any word in the sentence. Dangling modifiers are easy to repair, but they can be hard to recognize, especially in your own writing.

Recognizing dangling modifiers

Dangling modifiers are usually word groups (such as verbal phrases) that suggest but do not name an actor. When a sentence opens with such a modifier, readers expect the subject of the next clause to name the actor. If it doesn't, the modifier dangles.

▶ *When the driver opened*
~~Opening~~ the window to let out a huge bumblebee, the car accidentally swerved into an oncoming car.

The car didn't open the window; the driver did.

▶ After completing seminary training, ~~women's~~ *women have often been denied* access to the pulpit. ~~has often been denied.~~

The women (not their access to the pulpit) complete the training.

The following sentences illustrate four common kinds of dangling modifiers.

DANGLING *Deciding to join the navy,* the recruiter enthusiastically pumped Joe's hand. [Participial phrase]

DANGLING *Upon entering the doctor's office,* a skeleton caught my attention. [Preposition followed by a gerund phrase]

DANGLING *To please the children,* some fireworks were set off a day early. [Infinitive phrase]

DANGLING *Though only sixteen,* UCLA accepted Martha's application. [Elliptical clause with an understood subject and verb]

These dangling modifiers falsely suggest that the recruiter decided to join the navy, that the skeleton entered the doctor's office, that the fireworks intended to please the children, and that UCLA is sixteen years old.

Checking for dangling modifiers

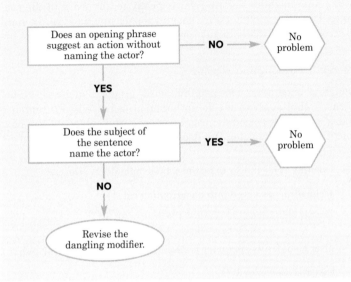

Although most readers will understand the writer's intended meaning in such sentences, the inadvertent humor can be distracting, and it can make the writer appear somewhat foolish.

ON THE WEB > dianahacker.com/writersref
Language Debates > Dangling modifiers

Repairing dangling modifiers

To repair a dangling modifier, you can revise the sentence in one of two ways:

1. Name the actor in the subject of the sentence, or
2. name the actor in the modifier.

Depending on your sentence, one of these revision strategies may be more appropriate than the other.

ACTOR NAMED IN SUBJECT

▶ Upon entering the doctor's office, a skeleton. ~~caught my attention.~~
                                              I noticed

▶ To please the children, some fireworks ~~were set off~~ a day early.
we set off

ACTOR NAMED IN MODIFIER

When Joe decided
▶ ~~Deciding~~ to join the navy, the recruiter enthusiastically
pumped ~~Joe's~~ hand.
his

Martha was
▶ Though only sixteen years old, UCLA accepted ~~Martha's~~
her
application.

NOTE: You cannot repair a dangling modifier just by moving it. Consider, for example, the sentence about the skeleton. If you put the modifier at the end of the sentence (*A skeleton caught my attention upon entering the doctor's office*), you are still suggesting—absurdly, of course—that the skeleton entered the office. The only way to avoid the problem is to put the word *I* in the sentence, either as the subject or in the modifier.

I noticed
▶ Upon entering the doctor's office, a skeleton. ~~caught my attention.~~

As I entered
▶ ~~Upon entering~~ the doctor's office, a skeleton caught my attention.

ON THE WEB > dianahacker.com/writersref
Grammar exercises > Sentence style > E-ex S3–1 through S3–4

S4

Shifts

GRAMMAR CHECKERS usually do not flag shifts in point of view or in verb tense, mood, or voice. Even obvious errors, like the following shift in tense, slip right past the grammar checker: *My three-year-old fell into the pool and to my surprise she swims to the shallow end.*

Sometimes grammar checkers mark a shift from direct to indirect question or quotation but do not make any suggestions for revision. You must decide where the structure is faulty and determine how to fix it.

S4-a Make the point of view consistent.

The point of view of a piece of writing is the perspective from which it is written: first person (*I* or *we*), second person (*you*), or third person (*he / she / it / one* or *they*).

The *I* (or *we*) point of view, which emphasizes the writer, is a good choice for informal letters and writing based primarily on personal experience. The *you* point of view, which emphasizes the reader, works well for giving advice or explaining how to do something. The third-person point of view, which emphasizes the subject, is appropriate in formal academic and professional writing.

Writers who are having difficulty settling on an appropriate point of view sometimes shift confusingly from one to another. The solution is to choose a suitable perspective and then stay with it.

▶ One week our class met in a junkyard to practice rescuing a victim trapped in a wrecked car. We learned to dismantle the car with the essential tools. ~~You~~ *We* were graded on ~~your~~ *our* speed and ~~your~~ *our* skill in extricating the victim.

The writer should have stayed with the *we* point of view. *You* is inappropriate because the writer is not addressing readers directly. *You* should not be used in a vague sense meaning "anyone." (See also G3-b.)

▶ ~~One needs~~ *You need* a password and a credit card number to access this database. You will be billed at an hourly rate.

You is an appropriate choice because the writer is giving advice directly to readers.

Shifts from the third-person singular to the third-person plural are especially common.

▶ ~~A police officer is~~ *Police officers are* often criticized for always being there when they aren't needed and never being there when they are.

Although the writer might have changed *they* to *he or she* (to match the singular *officer*), the revision in the plural is more concise. (See also G3-a.)

S4-b Maintain consistent verb tenses.

Consistent verb tenses clearly establish the time of the actions being described. When a passage begins in one tense and then shifts without warning and for no reason to another, readers are distracted and confused.

▶ There was no way I could fight the current. Just as I was losing
    jumped   *swam*
  hope, a stranger ~~jumps~~ off a passing boat and ~~swims~~ toward me.
              ^   ^

Writers often encounter difficulty with verb tenses when writing about literature. Because fictional events occur outside the time frames of real life, the past and the present tenses may seem equally appropriate. The literary convention, however, is to describe fictional events consistently in the present tense. (See also G2-f.)

▶ The scarlet letter is a punishment sternly placed on Hester's
                                              is
  breast by the community, and yet it ~~was~~ an extremely fanciful and
                                          ^
  imaginative product of Hester's own needlework.

S4-c Make verbs consistent in mood and voice.

Unnecessary shifts in the mood of a verb can be as distracting as needless shifts in tense. There are three moods in English: the indicative, used for facts, opinions, and questions; the imperative, used for orders or advice; and the subjunctive, used for wishes or conditions contrary to fact. (See G2-g.)

The following passage shifts confusingly from the indicative to the imperative mood.

▶ The officers advised us not to allow anyone into our homes
                                  They also suggested that we
  without proper identification. ~~Also,~~ alert neighbors to our
                                    ^
  vacation schedules.

Since the writer's purpose was to report the officers' advice, the revision puts both sentences in the indicative.

A verb may be in either the active voice (with the subject doing the action) or the passive voice (with the subject receiving the action). (See W3-a.) If a writer shifts without warning from one to the other, readers may be left wondering why.

▶ When the tickets are ready, the travel agent notifies the client/,
  lists each   *files*
  ~~Each~~ ticket ~~is then listed~~ on a daily register form, and a copy of

the itinerary. ~~is filed.~~

The passage began in the active voice (*agent notifies*) and then switched to the passive (*ticket is listed . . . copy is filed*). Because the active voice is clearer and more direct, the writer changed all the verbs to the active voice.

S4-d Avoid sudden shifts from indirect to direct questions or quotations.

An indirect question reports a question without asking it: *We asked whether we could visit Mimo.* A direct question asks directly: *Can we visit Mimo?* Sudden shifts from indirect to direct questions are awkward. In addition, sentences containing such shifts are impossible to punctuate because indirect questions must end with a period and direct questions must end with a question mark. (See P7-b.)

▶ I wonder whether Karla knew of the theft and, if so, ~~did~~
  whether she reported
  ~~she report~~ it to the police?.

The revision poses both questions indirectly. The writer could also ask both questions directly: *Did Karla know of the theft and, if so, did she report it to the police?*

An indirect quotation reports someone's words without quoting word for word: *Annabelle said that she is a Virgo.* A direct quotation presents the exact words of a speaker or writer, set off with quotation marks: *Annabelle said, "I am a Virgo."* Unannounced shifts from indirect to direct quotations are distracting and confusing, especially when the writer fails to insert the necessary quotation marks, as in the following example.

                                            asked me not to
▶ Mother said that she would be late for dinner and ~~please do not~~
                                came
  leave for choir practice until Dad ~~comes~~ home.

The revision reports all of the mother's words. The writer could also quote directly: *Mother said, "I will be late for dinner. Please do not leave for choir practice until Dad comes home."*

ON THE WEB > dianahacker.com/writersref
   Grammar exercises > Sentence style > E-ex S4–1 through S4–4

S5

Mixed constructions

A mixed construction contains elements that do not sensibly fit together. The mismatch may be a matter of grammar or of logic.

> GRAMMAR CHECKERS can flag *is when, is where,* and *reason . . . is because* constructions (S5-c), but they fail to identify nearly all other mixed constructions, including sentences as tangled as this one: *Depending on our method of travel and our destination determines how many suitcases we are allowed to pack.*

S5-a Untangle the grammatical structure.

Once you head into a sentence, your choices are limited by the range of grammatical patterns in English. (See B2 and B3.) You cannot begin with one grammatical plan and switch without warning to another.

MIXED   For most drivers who have a blood alcohol level of .05 percent double their risk of causing an accident.

REVISED   For most drivers who have a blood alcohol level of .05 percent, the risk of causing an accident is doubled.

REVISED   Most drivers who have a blood alcohol level of .05 percent double their risk of causing an accident.

The writer began with a long prepositional phrase that was destined to be a modifier but then tried to press it into service as the subject of the sentence. A prepositional phrase cannot serve as the subject of a sentence. If the sentence is to begin with the prepositional phrase, the writer must finish the sentence with a subject and verb (*risk . . . is doubled*). The writer who wishes to stay with the original verb (*double*) must head into the sentence another way (*Most drivers . . .*).

▶ *Being*
~~When an employee is~~ promoted without warning can be exciting
　　　^

or alarming.

The adverb clause *When an employee is promoted without warning*
cannot serve as the subject of the sentence. The revision replaces the
adverb clause with a gerund phrase, a word group that can function as
the subject. (See B3-b and B3-e.)

▶ Although the United States is one of the wealthiest nations

in the world, ~~but~~ more than 12 million of our children live in

poverty.

The *Although* clause is subordinate, so it cannot be linked to an independent clause with the coordinating conjunction *but.* (If you speak
English as a second language, see also E2-e.)

Occasionally a mixed construction is so tangled that it defies
grammatical analysis. When this happens, back away from the
sentence, rethink what you want to say, and then say it again as
clearly as you can.

MIXED　　In the whole-word method children learn to recognize
entire words rather than by the phonics method in
which they learn to sound out letters and groups of
letters.

REVISED　　The whole-word method teaches children to recognize
entire words; the phonics method teaches them to sound
out letters and groups of letters.

ESL　　English does not allow double subjects, nor does it allow an object or
an adverb to be repeated in an adjective clause. See E2-c and E2-d.
Unlike some languages, English does not allow a noun and a pronoun to be repeated in a sentence if they serve the same grammatical purpose. See E2-c.

▶ My father ~~he~~ moved to North Carolina before he met my

mother.

　　　　　　　　　　　　　　　　　the final exam
▶ ~~The final exam~~ I should really study for ~~it~~ to pass
　　　　　　　　　　　　　　　　^

the course.

S5-b Straighten out the logical connections.

The subject and the predicate should make sense together. When they don't, the error is known as *faulty predication*.

> ► Reluctantly we decided that ~~Tiffany's welfare~~ ^Tiffany^ would not be safe
>
> living with her mother.

Tiffany, not her welfare, may not be safe.

> ► Under the revised plan, the elderly ^double personal exemption for the^ ~~who now receive a double~~
>
> ~~personal exemption,~~ will be abolished.

The exemption, not the elderly, will be abolished.

An appositive and the noun to which it refers should be logically equivalent. When they are not, the error is known as *faulty apposition.*

> ► ~~The tax accountant,~~ ^Tax accounting,^ a very lucrative field, requires intelligence,
>
> patience, and attention to detail.

The tax accountant is a person, not a field.

S5-c Avoid *is when, is where,* and *reason . . . is because* constructions.

In formal English, many readers object to *is when, is where,* and *reason . . . is because* constructions on either logical or grammatical grounds.

> ► Anorexia nervosa is ^a disorder suffered by people who,^ ~~where people,~~ believing they are too fat, diet
>
> to the point of starvation.

Anorexia nervosa is a disorder, not a place.

> ► ~~The reason~~ I was late ~~is~~ because my motorcycle broke down.

The writer might have replaced the word *because* with *that,* but the preceding revision is more concise.

ON THE WEB > dianahacker.com/writersref
Grammar exercises > Sentence style > E-ex S5–1 and S5–2

S6

Sentence emphasis

Within each sentence, emphasize your point by expressing it in the subject and verb of an independent clause, the words that receive the most attention from readers (see S6-a to S6-e).

Within longer stretches of prose, you can draw attention to ideas deserving special emphasis by using a variety of techniques, often involving an unusual twist or some element of surprise (see S6-f).

S6-a Coordinate equal ideas; subordinate minor ideas.

When combining two or more ideas in one sentence, you have two choices: coordination or subordination. Choose coordination to indicate that the ideas are equal or nearly equal in importance. Choose subordination to indicate that one idea is less important than another.

> ✓ GRAMMAR CHECKERS do not catch the problems with coordination and subordination discussed in this section. Not surprisingly, computer programs have no way of sensing the relative importance of ideas.

Coordination

Coordination draws attention equally to two or more ideas. To coordinate single words or phrases, join them with a coordinating conjunction or with a pair of correlative conjunctions (see S1-b). To coordinate independent clauses — word groups that could each stand alone as a sentence — join them with a comma and a coordinating conjunction or with a semicolon. The semicolon is often accompanied by a conjunctive adverb such as *moreover, therefore,* or *however* or by a transitional phrase such as *for example* or *in other words.* (For a longer list, see P3-b.)

> Grandmother lost her sight, but her hearing sharpened.

> Grandmother lost her sight; however, her hearing sharpened.

Subordination

To give unequal emphasis to two or more ideas, express the major idea in an independent clause and place any minor ideas in subordinate clauses or phrases. (See B3.) Subordinate clauses, which cannot stand alone, typically begin with one of the following subordinating conjunctions or relative pronouns.

after	before	unless	which
although	if	until	while
as	since	when	who
as if	that	where	whom
because	though	whether	whose

Deciding which idea to emphasize is not a matter of right and wrong but is determined by the meaning you intend. Consider the two ideas about Grandmother's sight and hearing.

Grandmother lost her sight. Her hearing sharpened.

If your purpose is to stress your grandmother's acute hearing rather than her blindness, subordinate the idea concerning her blindness.

As Grandmother lost her sight, her hearing sharpened.

To focus on your grandmother's blindness, subordinate the idea about her hearing.

Though her hearing sharpened, Grandmother lost her sight.

S6-b Combine choppy sentences.

Short sentences demand attention, so you should use them primarily for emphasis. Too many short sentences, one after the other, make for a choppy style.

If an idea is not important enough to deserve its own sentence, try combining it with a sentence close by. Put any minor ideas in subordinate structures such as phrases or subordinate clauses. (See B3.)

▶ We keep our use of insecticides to a minimum/ ~~We~~ are concerned about their effect on the environment.

because we

A minor idea is now expressed in a subordinate clause beginning with *because.*

▶ ~~Sister Consilio was~~ $\overset{E}{\wedge}$nveloped in a black robe with only her face
and hands visible/, ~~She~~ $\underset{\wedge}{Sister\ Consilio}$ was an imposing figure.

A minor idea is now expressed in a participial phrase beginning with
Enveloped. (See B3-b.)

▶ My sister owes much of her recovery to a bodybuilding program/
$\underset{\wedge}{that\ she}$
~~She~~ began ~~the program~~ three years ago.

A minor idea is now expressed in an adjective clause beginning with
that. (See B3-e.)

ESL Unlike Arabic, Farsi, and other languages, English does not repeat
objects or adverbs in adjective clauses. The relative pronoun (*that,
which, whom*) or relative adverb (*where*) in the adjective clause rep-
resents the object or adverb. See E2-d.

▶ The apartment that we rented ~~it~~ needed repairs.

The pronoun *it* cannot repeat the relative pronoun *that*.

▶ The small town where my grandfather was born ~~there~~ is now

a big city.

The adverb *there* cannot repeat the relative adverb *where*.

Although subordination is ordinarily the most effective technique for combining short, choppy sentences, coordination is appropriate when the ideas are equal in importance.

▶ The hospital decides when patients will sleep and wake/, ~~It~~ dictates
$\overset{and}{\wedge}$
what and when they will eat/, ~~It~~ tells them when they may be with
$\wedge$
family and friends.

Equivalent ideas are expressed as parallel elements of a compound
predicate: *decides . . . dictates . . . tells.*

ON THE WEB > dianahacker.com/writersref
Grammar exercises > Sentence style > E-ex S6–1 and S6–2

S6-c Avoid ineffective coordination.

Coordinate structures are appropriate only when you intend to draw the reader's attention equally to two or more ideas: *Professor Sakellarios praises loudly, and she criticizes softly.* If one idea is more important than another—or if a coordinating conjunction does not clearly signal the relation between the ideas—you should subordinate the lesser idea.

▶ *After four hours,*
~~Four hours went by, and~~ a rescue truck finally arrived, but
   ^

by that time the injured swimmer had been evacuated in a

helicopter.

Three independent clauses were excessive. The least important idea has become a prepositional phrase. (See B3-a.)

S6-d Do not subordinate major ideas.

If a sentence buries its major idea in a subordinate construction, readers may not give the idea enough attention. Express the major idea in an independent clause and subordinate any minor ideas.

▶ Lanie, who now walks with the help of braces*had polio as a child,*/. ~~had polio as a~~
                                              ^   ^
~~child.~~

The writer wanted to focus on Lanie's ability to walk, but the original sentence buried this idea in an adjective clause. The revision puts the major idea in an independent clause and tucks the less important idea into an adjective clause (*who had polio as a child*). (See B3-e.)

▶ My uncle, *noticing* ~~noticed~~ my frightened look, ~~and~~ told me that the
            ^   ^

dentures in the glass were not real teeth.

The less important idea has become a participial phrase modifying the noun *uncle*.

ON THE WEB > dianahacker.com/writersref
Grammar exercises > Sentence style > E-ex S6–3

S6-e Do not subordinate excessively.

In attempting to avoid short, choppy sentences, writers sometimes move to the opposite extreme, putting more subordinate ideas into a sentence than its structure can bear. If a sentence collapses of its own weight, occasionally it can be restructured. More often, however, such sentences must be divided.

▶ Our job is to stay between the stacker and the tie machine

watching to see if the newspapers jam, *If they do,* ~~in which case~~ we pull the

bundles off and stack them on a skid, because otherwise they

would back up in the stacker.

S6-f Experiment with techniques for gaining special emphasis.

By experimenting with certain techniques, usually involving some element of surprise, you can draw attention to ideas that deserve special emphasis. Use such techniques sparingly, however, or they will lose their punch. The writer who tries to emphasize everything ends up emphasizing nothing.

Using sentence endings for emphasis

You can highlight an idea simply by withholding it until the end of a sentence. The technique works something like a punch line. In the following example, the sentence's meaning is not revealed until its very last word.

> The only completely consistent people are the dead.
> —Aldous Huxley

Using parallel structure for emphasis

Parallel grammatical structure draws special attention to paired ideas or to items in a series. (See S1.) When parallel ideas are paired, the emphasis falls on words that underscore comparisons or contrasts, especially when they occur at the end of a phrase or clause.

> We must *stop talking* about the *American dream* and *start listening* to the *dreams of Americans.*
> —Reubin Askew

In a parallel series, the emphasis falls at the end, so it is generally best to end with the most dramatic or climactic item in the series.

> Sister Charity enjoyed passing out writing punishments: translate the Ten Commandments into Latin, type a thousand-word essay on good manners, copy the New Testament with a quill pen.
>
> —Marie Visosky, student

Using an occasional short sentence for emphasis

Too many short sentences in a row will fast become monotonous (see S6-b), but an occasional short sentence, when played off against longer sentences in the same passage, will draw attention to an idea.

> The great secret, known to internists and learned early in marriage by internists' wives [or husbands], but still hidden from the general public, is that most things get better by themselves. Most things, in fact, are better by morning. —Lewis Thomas

S7

Sentence variety

When a rough draft is filled with too many same-sounding sentences, try to inject some variety—as long as you can do so without sacrificing clarity or ease of reading.

> GRAMMAR CHECKERS are of little help with sentence variety. It takes a human ear to know when and why sentence variety is needed.
>
> Some programs tell you when you have used the same word to open several sentences, but sometimes it is a good idea to do so—if you are trying to highlight parallel ideas, for example (see p. 33).

S7-a Use a variety of sentence structures.

A writer should not rely too heavily on simple sentences and compound sentences, for the effect tends to be both monotonous and choppy. (See S6-a and S6-b.) Too many complex sentences, however, can be equally monotonous. If your style tends to one or the other extreme, try to achieve a better mix of sentence types.

For a discussion of sentence types, see B4-a.

S7-b Use a variety of sentence openings.

Most sentences in English begin with the subject, move to the verb, and continue to an object, with modifiers tucked in along the way or put at the end. For the most part, such sentences are fine. Put too many of them in a row, however, and they become monotonous. Adverbial modifiers, being easily movable, can often be inserted at the beginning of the sentence, ahead of the subject. Such modifiers might be single words, phrases, or clauses.

▶ A few drops of sap ~~eventually~~ began to trickle from the tree
   Eventually a
   into the pail.

▶ A pair of black ducks flew over the lake. ~~just as the sun was~~
   Just as the sun was coming up, a
   ~~coming up~~.

For variety, adjectives and participial phrases can frequently be moved to the beginning of a sentence without loss of clarity. (See B3-b.)

▶ Edward/ ~~dejected and withdrawn,~~ nearly gave up his search
   Dejected and withdrawn,
   for a job.

▶ ~~Roberto and I,~~ anticipating a peaceful evening, sat cross-legged
   A   *Roberto and I*
   at the campfire to brew a cup of coffee and plan the rest of
   our hike.

TIP: When beginning a sentence with a participial phrase, make sure that the subject of the sentence names the person or thing described in the introductory phrase. If it doesn't, the phrase will dangle. (See S3-e.)

S7-c Try inverting sentences occasionally.

A sentence is inverted if it does not follow the normal subject-verb-object pattern. Many inversions sound artificial and should be avoided except in the most formal contexts. But if an inversion sounds natural, it can provide a welcome touch of variety.

Opposite the produce section is a

▶ A̬ refrigerated case of mouth-watering cheeses, ̬is opposite the

~~produce section.~~

Set at the top two corners of the stage were huge

▶ H̬uge lavender hearts outlined in bright white lights, ̬were set at

~~the top two corners of the stage.~~

W

Word Choice

W Word Choice

W 1

Glossary of usage

This glossary includes words commonly confused (such as *accept* and *except*), words commonly misused (such as *aggravate*), and words that are nonstandard (such as *hisself*). It also lists colloquialisms and jargon. Colloquialisms are expressions that may be appropriate in informal speech but are inappropriate in formal writing. Jargon is needlessly technical or pretentious language that is inappropriate in most contexts. If an item is not listed here, consult the index. For irregular verbs (such as *sing, sang, sung*), see G2-a. For idiomatic use of prepositions, see W5-d.

> ✓ GRAMMAR CHECKERS can point out commonly confused words and suggest that you check your usage. It is up to you, however, to determine the correct word for your intended meaning.

ON THE WEB > dianahacker.com/writersref
Language Debates > Absolute concepts such as *unique*
    bad versus *badly*
    however at the beginning of a sentence
    lie versus *lay*
    myself
    that versus *which*
    who versus *which* or *that*
    who versus *whom*
    you

a, an Use *an* before a vowel sound, *a* before a consonant sound: *an apple, a peach*. Problems sometimes arise with words beginning with *h* or *u*. If the *h* is silent, the word begins with a vowel sound, so use *an: an hour, an honorable deed*. If the *h* is pronounced, the word begins with a consonant sound, so use *a: a hospital, a historian, a hotel*. Words such as *university* and *union* begin with a consonant sound (a *y* sound), so use *a: a union*. Words such as *uncle* and *umbrella* begin with a vowel sound, so use *an: an underground well*. When an abbreviation or an acronym begins with a vowel sound, use *an: an EKG, an MRI, an AIDS patient*.

accept, except *Accept* is a verb meaning "to receive." *Except* is usually a preposition meaning "excluding." *I will accept all the packages except that one. Except* is also a verb meaning "to exclude." *Please except that item from the list.*

adapt, adopt   *Adapt* means "to adjust or become accustomed"; it is usually followed by *to. Adopt* means "to take as one's own." *Our family adopted a Vietnamese orphan, who quickly adapted to his new life.*

adverse, averse   *Adverse* means "unfavorable." *Averse* means "opposed" or "reluctant"; it is usually followed by *to. I am averse to your proposal because it could have an adverse impact on the economy.*

advice, advise   *Advice* is a noun, *advise* a verb. *We advise you to follow John's advice.*

affect, effect   *Affect* is usually a verb meaning "to influence." *Effect* is usually a noun meaning "result." *The drug did not affect the disease, and it had adverse side effects. Effect* can also be a verb meaning "to bring about." *Only the president can effect such a dramatic change.*

aggravate   *Aggravate* means "to make worse or more troublesome." *Overgrazing aggravated the soil erosion.* In formal writing, avoid the colloquial use of *aggravate* meaning "to annoy or irritate." *Her babbling annoyed* (not *aggravated*) *me.*

agree to, agree with   *Agree to* means "to give consent." *Agree with* means "to be in accord" or "to come to an understanding." *He agrees with me about the need for change, but he won't agree to my plan.*

ain't   *Ain't* is nonstandard. Use *am not, are not* (*aren't*), or *is not* (*isn't*). *I am not* (not *ain't*) *going home for spring break.*

all ready, already   *All ready* means "completely prepared." *Already* means "previously." *Susan was all ready for the concert, but her friends had already left.*

all right   *All right* is written as two words. *Alright* is nonstandard.

all together, altogether   *All together* means "everyone gathered." *Altogether* means "entirely." *We were not altogether certain that we could bring the family all together for the reunion.*

allude   To *allude* to something is to make an indirect reference to it. Do not use *allude* to mean "to refer directly." *In his lecture the professor referred* (not *alluded*) *to several pre-Socratic philosophers.*

allusion, illusion   An *allusion* is an indirect reference. An *illusion* is a misconception or false impression. *Did you catch my allusion to Shakespeare? Mirrors give the room an illusion of depth.*

a lot   *A lot* is two words. Do not write *alot. Sam lost a lot of weight.*

among, between   See *between, among.*

amongst   In American English, *among* is preferred.

amoral, immoral *Amoral* means "neither moral nor immoral"; it also means "not caring about moral judgments." *Immoral* means "morally wrong." *Until recently, most business courses were taught from an amoral perspective. Murder is immoral.*

amount, number Use *amount* with quantities that cannot be counted; use *number* with those that can. *This recipe calls for a large amount of sugar. We have a large number of toads in our garden.*

an See *a, an.*

and etc. *Et cetera* (*etc.*) means "and so forth," so *and etc.* is redundant. See also *etc.*

and/or Avoid the awkward construction *and/or* except in technical or legal documents.

angry at, angry with To write that one is *angry at* another person is nonstandard. Use *angry with* instead.

ante-, anti- The prefix *ante-* means "earlier" or "in front of"; the prefix *anti-* means "against" or "opposed to." *William Lloyd Garrison was a leader of the antislavery movement during the antebellum period.* *Anti-* should be used with a hyphen when it is followed by a capital letter or a word beginning with *i.*

anxious *Anxious* means "worried" or "apprehensive." In formal writing, avoid using *anxious* to mean "eager." *We are eager* (not *anxious*) *to see your new house.*

anybody, anyone *Anybody* and *anyone* are singular. (See G1-e and G3-a.)

anymore Reserve the adverb *anymore* for negative contexts, where it means "any longer." *Moviegoers are rarely shocked anymore by profanity.* Do not use *anymore* in positive contexts. Use *now* or *nowadays* instead. *Interest rates are so low nowadays* (not *anymore*) *that more people can afford to buy homes.*

anyone See *anybody, anyone.*

anyone, any one *Anyone,* an indefinite pronoun, means "any person at all." *Any one,* the pronoun *one* preceded by the adjective *any,* refers to a particular person or thing in a group. *Anyone from Chicago may choose any one of the games on display.*

anyplace In formal writing, use *anywhere.*

anyways, anywheres *Anyways* and *anywheres* are nonstandard. Use *anyway* and *anywhere.*

as *As* is sometimes used to mean "because." But do not use it if there is any chance of ambiguity. *We canceled the picnic because* (not *as*) *it began raining. As* here could mean "because" or "when."

as, like See *like, as.*

as to　*As to* is jargon for *about. He inquired about* (not *as to*) *the job.*

averse　See *adverse, averse.*

awful　The adjective *awful* and the adverb *awfully* are too colloquial for formal writing.

awhile, a while　*Awhile* is an adverb; it can modify a verb, but it cannot be the object of a preposition such as *for.* The two-word form *a while* is a noun preceded by an article and therefore can be the object of a preposition. *Stay awhile. Stay for a while.*

back up, backup　*Back up* is a verb phrase. *Back up the car carefully. Be sure to back up your hard drive. Backup* is a noun meaning "a duplicate of electronically stored data." *Keep your backup in a safe place. Backup* can also be used as an adjective. *I regularly create backup disks.*

bad, badly　*Bad* is an adjective, *badly* an adverb. (See G4-a and G4-b.) *They felt bad about being early and ruining the surprise. Her arm hurt badly after she slid headfirst into second base.*

being as, being that　*Being as* and *being that* are nonstandard expressions. Write *because* instead. *Because* (not *Being as*) *I slept late, I had to skip breakfast.*

beside, besides　*Beside* is a preposition meaning "at the side of" or "next to." *Annie Oakley slept with her gun beside her bed. Besides* is a preposition meaning "except" or "in addition to." *No one besides Terrie can have that ice cream. Besides* is also an adverb meaning "in addition." *I'm not hungry; besides, I don't like ice cream.*

between, among　Ordinarily, use *among* with three or more entities, *between* with two. *The prize was divided among several contestants. You have a choice between carrots and beans.*

bring, take　Use *bring* when an object is being transported toward you, *take* when it is being moved away. *Please bring me a glass of water. Please take these flowers to Mr. Scott.*

burst, bursted; bust, busted　*Burst* is an irregular verb meaning "to come open or fly apart suddenly or violently." Its principal parts are *burst, burst, burst.* The past-tense form *bursted* is nonstandard. *Bust* and *busted* are slang for *burst* and, along with *bursted,* should not be used in formal writing.

can, may　The distinction between *can* and *may* is fading, but some writers still observe it in formal writing. *Can* is traditionally reserved for ability, *may* for permission. *Can you speak French? May I help you?*

capital, capitol　*Capital* refers to a city, *capitol* to a building where lawmakers meet. *Capital* also refers to wealth or resources. *The capitol has undergone extensive renovations. The residents of the state capital protested the development plans.*

censor, censure   *Censor* means "to remove or suppress material considered objectionable." *Censure* means "to criticize severely." *The school's policy of censoring books has been censured by the media.*

cite, site   *Cite* means "to quote as an authority or example." *Site* is usually a noun meaning "a particular place." *He cited the zoning law in his argument against the proposed site of the gas station.* Locations on the Internet are usually referred to as *sites*. *The library's Web site improves every week.*

climactic, climatic   *Climactic* is derived from *climax*, the point of greatest intensity in a series or progression of events. *Climatic* is derived from *climate* and refers to meteorological conditions. *The climactic period in the dinosaurs' reign was reached just before severe climatic conditions brought on an ice age.*

coarse, course   *Coarse* means "crude" or "rough in texture." *The coarse weave of the wall hanging gave it a three-dimensional quality.* *Course* usually refers to a path, a playing field, or a unit of study; the expression *of course* means "certainly." *I plan to take a course in car repair this summer. Of course, you are welcome to join me.*

compare to, compare with   *Compare to* means "to represent as similar." *She compared him to a wild stallion.* *Compare with* means "to examine similarities and differences." *The study compared the language ability of apes with that of dolphins.*

complement, compliment   *Complement* is a verb meaning "to go with or complete" or a noun meaning "something that completes." *Compliment* as a verb means "to flatter"; as a noun it means "flattering remark." *Her skill at rushing the net complements his skill at volleying. Mother's flower arrangements receive many compliments.*

conscience, conscious   *Conscience* is a noun meaning "moral principles." *Conscious* is an adjective meaning "aware or alert." *Let your conscience be your guide. Were you conscious of his love for you?*

continual, continuous   *Continual* means "repeated regularly and frequently." *She grew weary of the continual telephone calls.* *Continuous* means "extended or prolonged without interruption." *The broken siren made a continuous wail.*

could care less   *Could care less* is a nonstandard expression. Write *couldn't care less* instead. *He couldn't* (not *could*) *care less about his psychology final.*

could of   *Could of* is nonstandard for *could have*. *We could have* (not *could of*) *taken the train.*

council, counsel   A *council* is a deliberative body, and a *councilor* is a member of such a body. *Counsel* usually means "advice" and can also mean "lawyer"; *counselor* is one who gives advice or guidance. *The* *councilors met to draft the council's position paper. The pastor offered wise counsel to the troubled teenager.*

criteria   *Criteria* is the plural of *criterion,* which means "a standard or rule or test on which a judgment or decision can be based." *The only criterion for the scholarship is ability.*

data   *Data* is a plural noun technically meaning "facts or propositions." But *data* is increasingly being accepted as a singular noun. *The new data suggest* (or *suggests*) *that our theory is correct.* (The singular *datum* is rarely used.)

different from, different than   Ordinarily, write *different from. Your sense of style is different from Jim's.* However, *different than* is acceptable to avoid an awkward construction. *Please let me know if your plans are different than* (to avoid *from what*) *they were six weeks ago.*

differ from, differ with   *Differ from* means "to be unlike"; *differ with* means "to disagree." *She differed with me about the wording of the agreement. My approach to the problem differed from hers.*

disinterested, uninterested   *Disinterested* means "impartial, objective"; *uninterested* means "not interested." *We sought the advice of a disinterested counselor to help us solve our problem. He was uninterested in anyone's opinion but his own.*

don't   *Don't* is the contraction for *do not. I don't want any. Don't* should not be used as the contraction for *does not,* which is *doesn't. He doesn't* (not *don't*) *want any.*

due to   *Due to* is an adjective phrase and should not be used as a preposition meaning "because of." *The trip was canceled because of* (not *due to*) *lack of interest. Due to* is acceptable as a subject complement and usually follows a form of the verb *be. His success was due to hard work.*

each   *Each* is singular. (See G1-e and G3-a.)

effect   See *affect, effect.*

e.g.   In formal writing, replace the Latin abbreviation *e.g.* with its English equivalent: *for example* or *for instance.*

either   *Either* is singular. (See G1-e and G3-a.) For *either . . . or* constructions, see G1-d and G3-a.

elicit, illicit   *Elicit* is a verb meaning "to bring out" or "to evoke." *Illicit* is an adjective meaning "unlawful." *The reporter was unable to elicit any information from the police about illicit drug traffic.*

emigrate from, immigrate to   *Emigrate* means "to leave one country or region to settle in another." *In 1900, my grandfather emigrated from Russia to escape the religious pogroms. Immigrate* means "to enter another country and reside there." *Many Mexicans immigrate to the United States to find work.*

eminent, imminent *Eminent* means "outstanding" or "distinguished." *We met an eminent professor of Greek history. Imminent* means "about to happen." *The announcement is imminent.*

enthused Many people object to the use of *enthused* as an adjective. Use *enthusiastic* instead. *The children were enthusiastic* (not *enthused*) *about going to the circus.*

etc. Avoid ending a list with *etc.* It is more emphatic to end with an example, and in most contexts readers will understand that the list is not exhaustive. When you don't wish to end with an example, *and so on* is more graceful than *etc.*

eventually, ultimately Often used interchangeably, *eventually* is the better choice to mean "at an unspecified time in the future" and *ultimately* is better to mean "the furthest possible extent or greatest extreme." *He knew that eventually he would complete his degree. The existentialist considered suicide the ultimately rational act.*

everybody, everyone *Everybody* and *everyone* are singular. (See G1-e and G3-a.)

everyone, every one *Everyone* is an indefinite pronoun. *Every one,* the pronoun *one* preceded by the adjective *every,* means "each individual or thing in a particular group." *Every one* is usually followed by *of. Everyone wanted to go. Every one of the missing books was found.*

except See *accept, except.*

expect Avoid the colloquial use of *expect* meaning "to believe, think, or suppose." *I think* (not *expect*) *it will rain tonight.*

explicit, implicit *Explicit* means "expressed directly" or "clearly defined"; *implicit* means "implied, unstated." *I gave him explicit instructions not to go swimming. My mother's silence indicated her implicit approval.*

farther, further *Farther* usually describes distances. *Further* usually suggests quantity or degree. *Chicago is farther from Miami than I thought. You extended the curfew further than you should have.*

fewer, less *Fewer* refers to items that can be counted; *less* refers to items that cannot be counted. *Fewer people are living in the city. Please put less sugar in my tea.*

finalize *Finalize* is jargon meaning "to make final or complete." Use ordinary English instead. *The architect prepared final drawings* (not *finalized the drawings*).

firstly *Firstly* sounds pretentious, and it leads to the ungainly series *firstly, secondly, thirdly,* and so on. Write *first, second, third* instead.

further See *farther, further.*

get   *Get* has many colloquial uses. In writing, avoid using *get* to mean the following: "to evoke an emotional response" (*That music always gets to me*); "to annoy" (*After a while his sulking got to me*); "to take revenge on" (*I got back at him by leaving the room*); "to become" (*He got sick*); "to start or begin" (*Let's get going*). Avoid using *have got to* in place of *must*. *I must* (not *have got to*) *finish this paper tonight.*

good, well   *Good* is an adjective, *well* an adverb. (See G4.) *He hasn't felt good about his game since he sprained his wrist last season. She performed well on the uneven parallel bars.*

graduate   Both of the following uses of *graduate* are standard: *My sister was graduated from UCLA last year. My sister graduated from UCLA last year.* It is nonstandard, however, to drop the word *from*: *My sister graduated UCLA last year.* Though this usage is common in informal English, many readers object to it.

grow   Phrases such as *to grow the economy* and *to grow a business* are jargon. Usually the verb *grow* is intransitive (it does not take a direct object). *Our business has grown very quickly.* When *grow* is used in a transitive sense, with a direct object, it means "to cultivate" or "to allow to grow." *We plan to grow tomatoes this year. John is growing a beard.*

hanged, hung   *Hanged* is the past-tense and past-participle form of the verb *hang* meaning "to execute." *The prisoner was hanged at dawn. Hung* is the past-tense and past-participle form of the verb *hang* meaning "to fasten or suspend." *The stockings were hung by the chimney with care.*

hardly   Avoid expressions such as *can't hardly* and *not hardly,* which are considered double negatives. *I can* (not *can't*) *hardly describe my elation at getting the job.* (See G4-d.)

has got, have got   *Got* is unnecessary and awkward in such constructions. It should be dropped. *We have* (not *have got*) *three days to prepare for the opening.*

he   At one time *he* was commonly used to mean "he or she." Today such usage is inappropriate. (See W4-e and G3-a.)

he/she, his/her   In formal writing, use *he or she* or *his or her.* For alternatives to these wordy constructions, see W4-e and G3-a.

hisself   *Hisself* is nonstandard. Use *himself.*

hopefully   *Hopefully* means "in a hopeful manner." *We looked hopefully to the future.* Some usage experts object to the use of *hopefully* as a sentence adverb, apparently on grounds of clarity. To be safe, avoid using *hopefully* in sentences such as the following: *Hopefully, your son will recover soon.* At least some educated readers will want you to indicate who is doing the hoping: *I hope that your son will recover soon.*

however   In the past, some writers objected to *however* at the beginning of a sentence, but current experts advise you to place the word according to your meaning and desired emphasis. Any of the following sentences is correct, depending on the intended contrast. *Pam decided, however, to attend Harvard. However, Pam decided to attend Harvard.* (She had been considering other schools.) *Pam, however, decided to attend Harvard.* (Unlike someone else, Pam opted for Harvard.)

hung See *hanged, hung.*

i.e. In formal writing, replace the Latin abbreviation *i.e.* with its English equivalent: *that is.*

if, whether Use *if* to express a condition and *whether* to express alternatives. *If you go on a trip, whether to Nebraska or New Jersey, remember to bring traveler's checks.*

illusion See *allusion, illusion.*

immigrate See *emigrate from, immigrate to.*

imminent See *eminent, imminent.*

immoral See *amoral, immoral.*

implement *Implement* is a pretentious way of saying "do," "carry out," or "accomplish." Use ordinary language instead. *We carried out* (not *implemented) the director's orders with some reluctance.*

imply, infer *Imply* means "to suggest or state indirectly"; *infer* means "to draw a conclusion." *John implied that he knew all about computers, but the interviewer inferred that John was inexperienced.*

in, into *In* indicates location or condition; *into* indicates movement or a change in condition. *They found the lost letters in a box after moving into the house.*

in regards to *In regards to* confuses two different phrases: *in regard to* and *as regards.* Use one or the other. *In regard to* (or *As regards) the contract, ignore the first clause.*

irregardless *Irregardless* is nonstandard. Use *regardless.*

is when, is where These mixed constructions are often incorrectly used in definitions. *A run-off election is a second election held to break a tie* (not *is when a second election breaks a tie*). (See S5-c.)

its, it's *Its* is a possessive pronoun; *it's* is a contraction for *it is.* (See P5-c and P5-e.) *The dog licked its wound whenever its owner walked into the room. It's a perfect day to walk the twenty-mile trail.*

kind(s) *Kind* is singular and should be treated as such. Don't write *These kind of chairs are rare.* Write instead *This kind of chair is rare. Kinds* is plural and should be used only when you mean more than one kind. *These kinds of chairs are rare.*

kind of, sort of Avoid using *kind of* or *sort of* to mean "somewhat." *The movie was somewhat* (not *kind of*) *boring.* Do not put *a* after either phrase. *That kind of* (not *kind of a*) *salesclerk annoys me.*

lay, lie See *lie, lay.*

lead, led *Lead* is a metallic element; it is a noun. *Led* is the past tense of the verb *lead. He led me to the treasure.*

learn, teach *Learn* means "to gain knowledge"; *teach* means "to impart knowledge." *I must teach* (not *learn*) *my sister to read.*

leave, let *Leave* means "to exit." Avoid using it with the nonstandard meaning "to permit." *Let* (not *Leave*) *me help you with the dishes.*

less See *fewer, less.*

let, leave See *leave, let.*

liable *Liable* means "obligated" or "responsible." Do not use it to mean "likely." *You're likely* (not *liable*) *to trip if you don't tie your shoelaces.*

lie, lay *Lie* is an intransitive verb meaning "to recline or rest on a surface." Its principal parts are *lie, lay, lain. Lay* is a transitive verb meaning "to put or place." Its principal parts are *lay, laid, laid.* (See G2-b.)

like, as *Like* is a preposition, not a subordinating conjunction. It can be followed only by a noun or a noun phrase. *As* is a subordinating conjunction that introduces a subordinate clause. In casual speech you may say *She looks like she hasn't slept* or *You don't know her like I do.* But in formal writing, use *as. She looks as if she hasn't slept. You don't know her as I do.* (See also B1-f and B1-g.)

loose, lose *Loose* is an adjective meaning "not securely fastened." *Lose* is a verb meaning "to misplace" or "to not win." *Did you lose your only loose pair of work pants?*

lots, lots of *Lots* and *lots of* are colloquial substitutes for *many, much,* or *a lot.* Avoid using them in formal writing.

mankind Avoid *mankind* whenever possible. It offends many readers because it excludes women. Use *humanity, humans, the human race,* or *humankind* instead. (See W4-e.)

may See *can, may.*

maybe, may be *Maybe* is an adverb meaning "possibly." *May be* is a verb phrase. *Maybe the sun will shine tomorrow. Tomorrow may be a brighter day.*

may of, might of *May of* and *might of* are nonstandard for *may have* and *might have. We may have* (not *may of*) *had too many cookies.*

media, medium *Media* is the plural of *medium. Of all the media that cover the Olympics, television is the medium that best captures the spectacle of the events.*

most   *Most* is colloquial when used to mean "almost" and should be avoided. *Almost* (not *Most*) *everyone went to the parade.*

must of   See *may of.*

myself   *Myself* is a reflexive or intensive pronoun. Reflexive: *I cut myself.* Intensive: *I will drive you myself.* Do not use *myself* in place of *I* or *me. He gave the flowers to Melinda and me* (not *myself*). (See also G3-c.)

neither   *Neither* is singular. (See G1-e and G3-a.) For *neither . . . nor* constructions, see G1-d and G3-a.

none   *None* may be singular or plural. (See G1-e.)

nowheres   *Nowheres* is nonstandard for *nowhere.*

number   See *amount, number.*

of   Use the verb *have,* not the preposition *of,* after the verbs *could, should, would, may, might,* and *must. They must have* (not *must of*) *left early.*

off of   *Off* is sufficient. Omit *of. The ball rolled off* (not *off of*) *the table.*

OK, O.K., okay   All three spellings are acceptable, but in formal speech and writing avoid these colloquial expressions.

parameters   *Parameter* is a mathematical term that has become jargon for "fixed limit," "boundary," or "guideline." Use ordinary English instead. *The task force was asked to work within certain guidelines* (not *parameters*).

passed, past   *Passed* is the past tense of the verb *pass. Mother passed me another slice of cake. Past* usually means "belonging to a former time" or "beyond a time or place." *Our past president spoke until past midnight. The hotel is just past the next intersection.*

percent, per cent, percentage   *Percent* (also spelled *per cent*) is always used with a specific number. *Percentage* is used with a descriptive term such as *large* or *small,* not with a specific number. *The candidate won 80 percent of the primary vote. Only a small percentage of registered voters turned out for the election.*

phenomena   *Phenomena* is the plural of *phenomenon,* which means "an observable occurrence or fact." *Strange phenomena occur at all hours of the night in that house, but last night's phenomenon was the strangest of all.*

plus   *Plus* should not be used to join independent clauses. *This raincoat is dirty; moreover* (not *plus*), *it has a hole in it.*

precede, proceed   *Precede* means "to come before." *Proceed* means "to go forward." *As we proceeded up the mountain path, we noticed fresh tracks in the mud, evidence that a group of hikers had preceded us.*

principal, principle   *Principal* is a noun meaning "the head of a school or an organization" or "a sum of money." It is also an adjective meaning "most important." *Principle* is a noun meaning "a basic truth or law." *The principal expelled her for three principal reasons. We believe in the principle of equal justice for all.*

proceed, precede   See *precede, proceed.*

quote, quotation   *Quote* is a verb; *quotation* is a noun. Avoid using *quote* as a shortened form of *quotation. Her quotations* (not *quotes*) *from Shakespeare intrigued us.*

raise, rise   *Raise* is a transitive verb meaning "to move or cause to move upward." It takes a direct object. *I raised the shades. Rise* is an intransitive verb meaning "to go up." *Heat rises.*

real, really   *Real* is an adjective; *really* is an adverb. *Real* is sometimes used informally as an adverb, but avoid this use in formal writing. *She was really* (not *real*) *angry.* (See G4-a.)

reason . . . is because   Use *that* instead of *because. The reason she's cranky is that* (not *because*) *she didn't sleep last night.* (See S5-c.)

reason why   The expression *reason why* is redundant. *The reason* (not *The reason why*) *Jones lost the election is clear.*

relation, relationship   *Relation* describes a connection between things. *Relationship* describes a connection between people. *There is a relation between poverty and infant mortality. Our business relationship has cooled over the years.*

respectfully, respectively   *Respectfully* means "showing or marked by respect." *Respectively* means "each in the order given." *He respectfully submitted his opinion to the judge. John, Tom, and Larry were a butcher, a baker, and a lawyer, respectively.*

sensual, sensuous   *Sensual* means "gratifying the physical senses," especially those associated with sexual pleasure. *Sensuous* means "pleasing to the senses," especially those involved in the experience of art, music, and nature. *The sensuous music and balmy air led the dancers to more sensual movements.*

set, sit   *Set* is a transitive verb meaning "to put" or "to place." Its principal parts are *set, set, set. Sit* is an intransitive verb meaning "to be seated." Its principal parts are *sit, sat, sat. She set the dough in a warm corner of the kitchen. The cat sat in the warmest part of the room.*

shall, will   *Shall* was once used as the helping verb with *I* or *we: I shall, we shall, you will, he/she/it will, they will.* Today, however, *will* is generally accepted even when the subject is *I* or *we.* The word *shall* occurs primarily in polite questions (*Shall I find you a pillow?*) and in legalistic sentences suggesting duty or obligation (*The applicant shall file form 1080 by December 31*).

should of   *Should of* is nonstandard for *should have*. *They should have* (not *should of*) *been home an hour ago.*

since   Do not use *since* to mean "because" if there is any chance of ambiguity. *Because* (not *Since*) *we won the game, we have been celebrating with a pitcher of root beer. Since* here could mean "because" or "from the time that."

sit   See *set, sit.*

site   See *cite, site.*

somebody, someone   *Somebody* and *someone* are singular. (See G1-e and G3-a.)

something   *Something* is singular. (See G1-e.)

sometime, some time, sometimes   *Sometime* is an adverb meaning "at an indefinite or unstated time." *Some time* is the adjective *some* modifying the noun *time* and is spelled as two words to mean "a period of time." *Sometimes* is an adverb meaning "at times, now and then." *I'll see you sometime soon. I haven't lived there for some time. Sometimes I run into him at the library.*

suppose to   Write *supposed to.*

sure and   Write *sure to. We were all taught to be sure to* (not *and*) *look both ways before crossing a street.*

take   See *bring, take.*

than, then   *Than* is a conjunction used in comparisons; *then* is an adverb denoting time. *That pizza is more than I can eat. Tom laughed, and then we recognized him.*

that   See *who, which, that.*

that, which   Many writers reserve *that* for restrictive clauses, *which* for nonrestrictive clauses. (See P1-e.)

theirselves   *Theirselves* is nonstandard for *themselves. The crash victims pushed the car out of the way themselves* (not *theirselves*).

them   The use of *them* in place of *those* is nonstandard. *Please send those* (not *them*) *flowers to the patient in room 220.*

there, their, they're   *There* is an adverb specifying place; it is also an expletive. Adverb: *Sylvia is lying there unconscious.* Expletive: *There are two plums left. Their* is a possessive pronoun. *Fred and Jane finally washed their car. They're* is a contraction of *they are. They're later than usual today.*

they   The use of *they* to indicate possession is nonstandard. Use *their* instead. *Cindy and Sam decided to sell their* (not *they*) *1975 Corvette.*

this kind   See *kind(s).*

to, too, two   *To* is a preposition; *too* is an adverb; *two* is a number. *Too many of your shots slice to the left, but the last two were just right.*

toward, towards   *Toward* and *towards* are generally interchangeable, although *toward* is preferred in American English.

try and   *Try and* is nonstandard for *try to. The teacher asked us all to try to* (not *try and*) *write an original haiku.*

ultimately, eventually   See *eventually, ultimately.*

unique   Avoid expressions such as *most unique, more straight, less perfect, very round.* Either something is unique or it isn't. It is illogical to suggest degrees of uniqueness. (See G4-c.)

usage   The noun *usage* should not be substituted for *use* when the meaning is "employment of." *The use* (not *usage*) *of computers dramatically increased the company's profits.*

use to   Write *used to.*

utilize   *Utilize* means "to make use of." It often sounds pretentious; in most cases, *use* is sufficient. *I used* (not *utilized*) *the laser printer.*

wait for, wait on   *Wait for* means "to be in readiness for" or "await." *Wait on* means "to serve." *We're only waiting for* (not *waiting on*) *Ruth to take us to the game.*

ways   *Ways* is colloquial when used to mean "distance." *The city is a long way* (not *ways*) *from here.*

weather, whether   The noun *weather* refers to the state of the atmosphere. *Whether* is a conjunction referring to a choice between alternatives. *We wondered whether the weather would clear.*

well, good   See *good, well.*

where   Do not use *where* in place of *that. I heard that* (not *where*) *the crime rate is increasing.*

which   See *that, which* and *who, which, that.*

while   Avoid using *while* to mean "although" or "whereas" if there is any chance of ambiguity. *Although* (not *While*) *Gloria lost money in the slot machine, Tom won it at roulette.* Here *While* could mean either "although" or "at the same time that."

who, which, that   Do not use *which* to refer to persons. Use *who* instead. *That,* though generally used to refer to things, may be used to refer to a group or class of people. *The player who* (not *that* or *which*) *made the basket at the buzzer was named MVP. The team that scores the most points in this game will win the tournament.*

who, whom   *Who* is used for subjects and subject complements; *whom* is used for objects. (See G3-d.)

who's, whose *Who's* is a contraction of *who is; whose* is a possessive pronoun. *Who's ready for more popcorn? Whose coat is this?* (See P5-c and P5-e.)

will See *shall, will.*

would of *Would of* is nonstandard for *would have. She would have* (not *would of*) *had a chance to play if she had arrived on time.*

you In formal writing, avoid *you* in an indefinite sense meaning "anyone." (See G3-b.) *Any spectator* (not *You*) *could tell by the way John caught the ball that his throw would be too late.*

your, you're *Your* is a possessive pronoun; *you're* is a contraction of *you are. Is that your new motorcycle? You're on the list of finalists.* (See P5-c and P5-e.)

W2

Wordy sentences

Long sentences are not necessarily wordy, nor are short sentences always concise. A sentence is wordy if it can be tightened without loss of meaning.

> GRAMMAR CHECKERS flag wordy constructions only occasionally. They sometimes alert you to common redundancies, such as *true fact,* but they overlook more redundancies than they catch. They may miss empty or inflated phrases, such as *in my opinion* and *in order that,* and they rarely identify sentences with needlessly complex structures. Grammar checkers are very good, however, at flagging and suggesting revisions for wordy constructions beginning with *there is* and *there are.*

W2-a Eliminate redundancies.

Redundancies such as *cooperate together, close proximity, basic essentials,* and *true fact* are a common source of wordiness. There is no need to say the same thing twice.

▶ Daniel ~~is now employed~~ at a private rehabilitation center ~~working~~ *works*
  as a registered physical therapist.

Though modifiers ordinarily add meaning to the words they modify, occasionally they are redundant.

▶ Sylvia ~~very hurriedly~~ scribbled her name, address, and phone number on the back of a greasy napkin.

▶ Joel was determined ~~in his mind~~ to lose weight.

The words *scribbled* and *determined* already contain the notions suggested by the modifiers *very hurriedly* and *in his mind.*

W2-b Avoid unnecessary repetition of words.

Though words may be repeated deliberately, for effect, repetitions will seem awkward if they are clearly unnecessary. When a more concise version is possible, choose it.

▶ Our fifth patient, in room six, is ~~a~~ mentally ill ~~patient.~~

▶ The best teachers help each student to *grow* ~~become a better student~~ both academically and emotionally.

W2-c Cut empty or inflated phrases.

An empty phrase can be cut with little or no loss of meaning. Common examples are introductory word groups that apologize or hedge: *in my opinion, I think that, it seems that, one must admit that,* and so on.

▶ ~~In my opinion,~~ *O*ur current immigration policy is misguided.

Inflated phrases can be reduced to a word or two without loss of meaning.

INFLATED	CONCISE
along the lines of	like
as a matter of fact	in fact
at all times	always
at the present time	now, currently
at this point in time	now, currently

INFLATED	CONCISE
because of the fact that	because
by means of	by
due to the fact that	because
for the purpose of	for
for the reason that	because
have the ability to	can, be able to
in order to	to
in spite of the fact that	although, though
in the event that	if
in the final analysis	finally
in the nature of	like
in the neighborhood of	about
until such time as	until

► We will file the appropriate papers ~~in the event that~~ *if* we are

unable to meet the deadline.

W2-d Simplify the structure.

If the structure of a sentence is needlessly indirect, try simplifying it. Look for opportunities to strengthen the verb.

► The CEO claimed that because of volatile market conditions she

could not ~~make an~~ estimate ~~of~~ the company's future profits.

The verb *estimate* is more vigorous and more concise than *make an estimate of*.

The colorless verbs *is, are, was,* and *were* frequently generate excess words. (See also W3-b.)

► Eduartina ~~is responsible for monitoring and balancing~~ *monitors and balances* the

budgets for travel and personnel.

The revision is more direct and concise. Actions orginally appearing in subordinate structures have become verbs replacing *is*.

The expletive constructions *there is* and *there are* (or *there was* and *there were*) can also generate excess words. The same is true of expletive constructions beginning with *it*.

▶ ~~There is~~ ^A^ ~~a~~nother module ~~that~~ tells the story of Charles Darwin and introduces the theory of evolution.

▶ ~~It is imperative that~~ ^A^ ~~a~~ll police officers ^must^ follow strict procedures when apprehending a suspect.

Finally, verbs in the passive voice may be needlessly indirect. When the active voice expresses your meaning as well, use it. (See also W3-a.)

▶ All too often, ^our coaches have recruited^ athletes with marginal academic skills. ~~have been recruited by our coaches.~~

W2-e Reduce clauses to phrases, phrases to single words.

Word groups functioning as modifiers can often be made more compact. Look for any opportunities to reduce clauses to phrases or phrases to single words.

▶ We visited Monticello, ~~which was~~ the home of Thomas Jefferson.

▶ For her birthday we gave Jess a stylish vest, ^silk^ ~~made of silk.~~

ON THE WEB > dianahacker.com/writersref
Grammar exercises > Word choice > E-ex W2–1 through W2–3

W3

Active verbs

As a rule, choose an active verb and pair it with a subject that names the person or thing doing the action. Active verbs express meaning more emphatically and vigorously than their weaker counterparts—forms of the verb *be* or verbs in the passive voice.

Verbs in the passive voice lack strength because their subjects receive the action instead of doing it (see also B2-b). Forms of the verb *be* (*be, am, is, are, was, were, being, been*) lack vigor because they convey no action.

Although passive verbs and the forms of *be* have legitimate uses, if an active verb can carry your meaning, use it.

PASSIVE	The coolant pumps *were destroyed* by a surge of power.
BE VERB	A surge of power *was* responsible for the destruction of the coolant pumps.
ACTIVE	A surge of power *destroyed* the coolant pumps.

Even among active verbs, some are more active—and therefore more vigorous and colorful—than others. Carefully selected verbs can energize a piece of writing.

> ► The goalie crouched low, ~~reached~~ ^{swept} out his stick, and ~~sent~~ ^{hooked} the rebound away from the mouth of the net.

ACADEMIC ENGLISH Although you may be tempted to avoid the passive voice completely, keep in mind that it is preferred in some writing situations, especially in scientific writing. For appropriate uses of the passive voice, see W3-a; for advice about forming the passive, see E1-c.

GRAMMAR CHECKERS are fairly good at flagging passive verbs, such as *is used*. However, because passive verbs are sometimes appropriate, you—not the computer program—must decide whether to change a verb from passive to active. Grammar checkers tend to suggest revisions only when the passive sentence contains a *by* phrase (*Carbon dating is used by scientists to determine an object's approximate age*). Occasionally they make inappropriate suggestions for revision (*Scientists to determine an object's approximate age use carbon dating*). Only you can determine the most sensible word order for your sentence.

W3-a Use the active voice unless you have a good reason for choosing the passive.

In the active voice, the subject of the sentence does the action; in the passive voice, the subject receives the action. (See also B2-b.)

ACTIVE   Hernando *caught* the fly ball.

PASSIVE   The fly ball *was caught* by Hernando.

In passive sentences, the actor (in this case *Hernando*) frequently disappears from the sentence: *The fly ball was caught.*

In most cases, you will want to emphasize the actor, so you should use the active voice. To replace a passive verb with an active alternative, make the actor the subject of the sentence.

▶ A bolt of lightning struck the transformer.
  ~~The transformer was struck by a bolt of lightning.~~
  ^

The active verb (*struck*) makes the point more forcefully than the passive verb (*was struck*).

The passive voice is appropriate if you wish to emphasize the receiver of the action or to minimize the importance of the actor.

APPROPRIATE   Many native Hawaiians *are forced* to leave their
PASSIVE   beautiful beaches to make room for hotels and
               condominiums.

APPROPRIATE   As the time for harvest approaches, the tobacco
PASSIVE   plants *are sprayed* with a chemical to retard the
               growth of suckers.

The writer of the first sentence wished to emphasize the receivers of the action, Hawaiians. The writer of the second sentence wished to focus on the tobacco plants, not on the people spraying them.

In much scientific writing, the passive voice properly emphasizes the experiment or process being described, not the researcher.

APPROPRIATE   The solution *was heated* to the boiling point, and
PASSIVE   then it was reduced in volume by 50 percent.

ON THE WEB > dianahacker.com/writersref
Language Debates > Passive voice

W3-b Replace *be* verbs that result in dull or wordy sentences.

Not every *be* verb needs replacing. The forms of *be* (*be, am, is, are, was, were, being, been*) work well when you want to link a subject to a noun that clearly renames it or to an adjective that describes it: *History is a bucket of ashes. Scoundrels are always sociable.* (See B2-b.) And when used as helping verbs before present participles (*is flying, are disappearing*) to express ongoing action, *be* verbs are fine: *Derrick was plowing the field when his wife went into labor.* (See G2-f.)

If using a *be* verb makes a sentence needlessly dull or wordy, however, consider replacing it. Often a phrase following the verb will contain a word (such as *violation*) that suggests a more vigorous, active alternative (*violate*).

>   *violate*
> ► Burying nuclear waste in Antarctica would ~~be in violation of~~
>   ^
> an international treaty.

Violate is less wordy and more vigorous than *be in violation of.*

>   *resisted*
> ► When Rosa Parks ~~was resistant to~~ giving up her seat on the bus,
>   ^
> she became a civil rights hero.

Resisted is stronger than *was resistant to.*

GRAMMAR CHECKERS usually do not flag wordiness caused by *be* verbs: *is in violation of.* Only you can find ways to strengthen your sentences by using vigorous, active verbs in place of *be.*

ON THE WEB > dianahacker.com/writersref
Grammar exercises > Word choice > E-ex W3–1 through W3–3

W4

Appropriate language

Language is appropriate when it suits your subject, engages your audience, and blends naturally with your own voice.

W4-a Stay away from jargon.

Jargon is specialized language used among members of a trade, profession, or group. Use jargon only when readers will be familiar with it; even then, use it only when plain English will not do as well.

JARGON   For years the indigenous body politic of South Africa attempted to negotiate legal enfranchisement without result.

REVISED   For years the indigenous people of South Africa negotiated in vain for the right to vote.

Broadly defined, jargon includes puffed-up language designed more to impress readers than to inform them. The following are common examples from business, government, higher education, and the military, with plain English translations in parentheses.

ameliorate (improve)

commence (begin)

components (parts)

endeavor (try)

exit (leave)

facilitate (help)

factor (consideration, cause)

impact (v.) (affect)

indicator (sign)

optimal (best, most favorable)

parameters (boundaries, limits)

peruse (read, look over)

prior to (before)

utilize (use)

viable (workable)

Sentences filled with jargon are hard to read, and they are often wordy as well.

▶ All ~~employees functioning in the capacity of~~ work-study students *must prove that they are currently enrolled.* ~~are required to give evidence of current enrollment.~~

         begin   *improving*
▶ Mayor Summers will ~~commence~~ his term of office by ~~ameliorating~~ living conditions in *poor neighborhoods.* ~~economically deprived zones.~~

W4-b Avoid pretentious language, most euphemisms, and "doublespeak."

Hoping to sound profound or poetic, some writers embroider their thoughts with large words and flowery phrases, language that in fact sounds pretentious. Pretentious language is so ornate and often so wordy that it obscures the thought that lies beneath.

      parents become old,
▶ When our ~~progenitors reach their silver-haired and golden years,~~
       bury   *old-age*
we frequently ~~ensepulcher~~ them in homes ~~for senescent beings~~ as
        dead.
if they were already ~~among the deceased.~~

Euphemisms, nice-sounding words or phrases substituted for words thought to sound harsh or ugly, are sometimes appropriate. It is customary, for example, to say that a couple is "sleeping together" or that someone has "passed away." Most euphemisms, however, are needlessly evasive or even deceitful. Like pretentious language, they obscure the intended meaning.

EUPHEMISM	PLAIN ENGLISH
adult entertainment	pornography
preowned automobile	used car
economically deprived	poor
selected out	fired
negative savings	debts
strategic withdrawal	retreat or defeat
revenue enhancers	taxes
chemical dependency	drug addiction
downsize	lay off
correctional facility	prison

The term *doublespeak* applies to any deliberately evasive or deceptive language, including euphemisms. Doublespeak is especially common in politics, where missiles are named "Peacekeepers," airplane crashes are termed "uncontrolled contact with the ground," and a military retreat is described as "tactical redeployment." Business also gives us its share of doublespeak. When the manufacturer of a pacemaker writes that its product "may result in adverse health consequences in pacemaker-dependent patients as a result of sudden 'no output' failure," it takes an alert reader to grasp the message: The pacemaker might suddenly stop functioning and cause a heart attack or even death.

GRAMMAR CHECKERS rarely identify jargon and only occasionally flag pretentious language. Sometimes they flag language that is acceptable in academic writing. You should be alert to your own use of jargon and pretentious language and simplify it whenever possible. If your grammar checker continually questions language that is appropriate in an academic setting, check to see whether you can set the program to a formal style level.

W4-c In most contexts, avoid slang, regional expressions, and nonstandard English.

Slang is an informal and sometimes private vocabulary that expresses the solidarity of a group such as teenagers, rock musicians, or football fans; it is subject to more rapid change than standard English. For example, the slang teenagers use to express approval changes every few years; *cool, groovy, neat, awesome, phat,* and *sweet* have replaced one another within the last three decades. Sometimes slang becomes so widespread that it is accepted as standard vocabulary. *Jazz,* for example, started as slang but is now generally accepted to describe a style of music.

Although slang has a certain vitality, it is a code that not everyone understands, and it is very informal. Therefore, it is inappropriate in most written work.

▶ If we don't begin studying for the final, a whole semester's work ~~is~~
will be wasted.
~~going down the tubes.~~
^

disgust you.
▶ The government's "filth" guidelines for food will ~~gross you out.~~
^

Regional expressions are common to a group in a geographical area. *Let's talk with the bark off* (for *Let's speak frankly*) is an expression in the southern United States, for example. Regional expressions have the same limitations as slang and are therefore inappropriate in most writing.

turn on
▶ John was four blocks from the house before he remembered to ~~cut~~
^
the headlights. ~~on.~~
^

▶ I'm not ~~for~~ sure, but I think the dance has been postponed.

Standard English is the language used in all academic, business, and professional fields. Nonstandard English is spoken by people with a common regional or social heritage. Although nonstandard English may be appropriate when spoken within a close group, it is out of place in most formal and informal writing.

has
▶ The counselor ~~have~~ so many problems in her own life that she
^
doesn't
~~don't~~ know how to advise anyone else.
^

If you speak a nonstandard dialect, try to identify the ways in which your dialect differs from standard English. Look especially for the following features of nonstandard English, which commonly cause problems in writing:

> Misuse of verb forms such as *began* and *begun* (See G2-a.)
>
> Omission of *-s* endings on verbs (See G2-c.)
>
> Omission of *-ed* endings on verbs (See G2-d.)
>
> Omission of necessary verbs (See G2-e.)
>
> Double negatives (See G4-d.)

You might also scan the Glossary of Usage (W1), which alerts you to nonstandard words and expressions such as *ain't, could of, hisself, theirselves, them* (meaning "those"), *they* (meaning "their"), and so on.

W4-d Choose an appropriate level of formality.

In deciding on a level of formality, consider both your subject and your audience. Does the subject demand a dignified treatment, or is a relaxed tone more suitable? Will the audience be put off if you assume too close a relationship with them, or might you alienate them by seeming too distant?

For most college and professional writing, some degree of formality is appropriate. In a letter applying for a job, for example, it is a mistake to sound too breezy and informal.

TOO INFORMAL	I'd like to get that technician job you've got in the paper.
MORE FORMAL	I would like to apply for the technician position listed in the *Peoria Journal Star.*

Informal writing is appropriate for private letters, business correspondence between close associates, articles in popular magazines, and personal narratives. In such writing, formal language can seem out of place.

>   *began*
> ▶ Bob's pitching lesson ~~commenced~~ with his famous sucker
>   *which he threw*^
> pitch, ~~implemented~~ as a slow ball coming behind a fast windup.
>   ^

Formal words such as *commenced* and *implemented* clash with appropriate informal terms such as *sucker pitch* and *fast windup.*

> ✓ GRAMMAR CHECKERS rarely flag slang and informal language. They do, however, flag contractions. If your ear tells you that a contraction such as *isn't* or *doesn't* strikes the right tone, stay with it.

W4-e Avoid sexist language.

Sexist language is language that stereotypes or demeans men or women, usually women. Using nonsexist language is a matter of courtesy — of respect for and sensitivity to the feelings of others.

> ✓ GRAMMAR CHECKERS are good at flagging obviously sexist terms, such as *mankind* and *fireman*, but they do not flag language that might be demeaning to women (*woman doctor*) or stereotypical (referring to assistants as women and lawyers as men, for instance). They also have no way of identifying the generic use of *he* or *his* (*An obstetrician needs to be available to his patients anytime, day or night*). You must use your common sense to tell when a word or a construction is offensive.

ON THE WEB > dianahacker.com/writersref
Language Debates > Sexist language

Recognizing sexist language

Some sexist language is easy to recognize because it reflects genuine contempt for women: referring to a woman as a "chick," for example, or calling a lawyer a "lady lawyer," or saying in an advertisement, "If our new sports car were a lady, it would get its bottom pinched."

Other forms of sexist language are less blatant. The following practices, while they may not result from conscious sexism, reflect stereotypical thinking: referring to nurses as women and doctors as men, using different conventions when naming or identifying women and men, or assuming that all of one's readers are men.

STEREOTYPICAL LANGUAGE

After the nursing student graduates, *she* must face a difficult state board examination. [Not all nursing students are women.]

Running for city council are Jake Stein, an attorney, and *Mrs. Cynthia Jones*, a professor of English *and mother of three*. [The title *Mrs.* and the phrase *and mother of three* are irrelevant.]

Wives of senior government officials are required to report any gifts they receive that are valued at more than $100. [Not all senior government officials are men.]

Still other forms of sexist language result from outmoded traditions. The pronouns *he, him,* and *his,* for instance, were traditionally used to refer generically to persons of either sex.

GENERIC *HE* OR *HIS*

When a senior physician is harassed by managed care professionals, *he* may be tempted to leave the profession.

A journalist is stimulated by *his* deadline.

Today, however, such usage is widely viewed as sexist because it excludes women and encourages sex-role stereotyping—the view that men are somehow more suited than women to be doctors, journalists, and so on.

Like the pronouns *he, him,* and *his,* the nouns *man* and *men* were once used indefinitely to refer to persons of either sex. Current usage demands gender-neutral terms instead.

INAPPROPRIATE	APPROPRIATE
anchorman	anchor
chairman	chairperson, moderator, chair, head
clergyman	member of the clergy, minister, pastor
congressman	member of Congress, representative, legislator
fireman	firefighter
foreman	supervisor
mailman	mail carrier, postal worker, letter carrier
(to) man	to operate, to staff
mankind	people, humans
manpower	personnel
policeman	police officer
salesman	sales associate, sales representative
weatherman	weather forecaster, meteorologist
workman	worker, laborer

Revising sexist language

When revising sexist language, be sparing in your use of the wordy constructions *he or she* and *his or her*. Although these constructions are fine in small doses, they become awkward when repeated throughout an essay. A better revision strategy, many writers have discovered, is to write in the plural; yet another strategy is to recast the sentence so that the problem does not arise.

SEXIST

When a senior physician is harassed by managed care professionals, *he* may be tempted to leave the profession.

A journalist is stimulated by *his* deadline.

ACCEPTABLE BUT WORDY

When a senior physician is harassed by managed care professionals, *he or she* may be tempted to leave the profession.

A journalist is stimulated by *his or her* deadline.

BETTER: USING THE PLURAL

When senior *physicians* are harassed by managed care professionals, *they* may be tempted to leave the profession.

Journalists are stimulated by *their* deadlines.

BETTER: RECASTING THE SENTENCE

When harassed by managed care professionals, *a senior physician* may be tempted to leave the profession.

A journalist is stimulated by *a* deadline.

For more examples of these revision strategies, see G3-a.

ON THE WEB > dianahacker.com/writersref
Grammar exercises > Word choice > E-ex W4–2

W4-f Revise language that may offend groups of people.

Obviously it is impolite to use offensive terms such as *Polack* or *redneck*. But biased language can take more subtle forms. Because language evolves over time, names once thought acceptable may become offensive. When describing groups of people, choose names that the groups currently use to describe themselves.

▶ North Dakota takes its name from the ~~Indian~~ *Lakota* word meaning
  "friend" or "ally."

▶ Many ~~Oriental~~ *Asian* immigrants have recently settled in our small
  town in Tennessee.

Negative stereotypes (such as "drives like a teenager" or "haggard as an old crone") are of course offensive. But you should avoid stereotyping a person or a group even if you believe your generalization to be positive.

▶ It was no surprise that Greer, ~~a Chinese American,~~ *an excellent math and science student,* was selected
  for the honors chemistry program.

W5

Exact language

Two reference works (or their online equivalents) will help you find words to express your meaning exactly: a good dictionary, such as *The American Heritage Dictionary* or *Merriam-Webster's Collegiate Dictionary,* and a book of synonyms and antonyms such as *Roget's International Thesaurus.* (See W6.)

☑ GRAMMAR CHECKERS flag some nonstandard idioms, such as *comply to,* but few clichés. They do not identify commonly confused words, such as *principal* and *principle,* or misused word forms, such as *significance* and *significant.* You must be alert for such words and use your dictionary if you are unsure of the correct form. Grammar checkers are of little help with the other problems discussed in W5: choosing words with appropriate connotations, using concrete language, and using figures of speech appropriately.

W5-a Select words with appropriate connotations.

In addition to their strict dictionary meanings (or *denotations*), words have *connotations,* emotional colorings that affect how readers respond to them. The word *steel* denotes "made of or resembling commercial iron that contains carbon," but it also calls up a cluster of images associated with steel, such as the sensation of touching it. These associations give the word its connotations—cold, smooth, unbending.

If the connotation of a word does not seem appropriate for your purpose, your audience, or your subject matter, you should change the word. When a more appropriate synonym does not come quickly to mind, consult a dictionary or a thesaurus. (See W6.)

▶ The model was ~~skinny~~ *slender* and fashionable.

The connotation of the word *skinny* is too negative.

▶ As I covered the boats with marsh grass, the ~~perspiration~~ *sweat* I had worked up evaporated in the wind, and the cold morning air seemed even colder.

The term *perspiration* is too dainty for the context, which suggests vigorous exercise.

W5-b Prefer specific, concrete nouns.

Unlike general nouns, which refer to broad classes of things, specific nouns point to definite and particular items. *Film,* for example, names a general class, *fantasy film* names a narrower class, and *Lord of the Rings: Return of the King* is more specific still.

Unlike abstract nouns, which refer to qualities and ideas (*justice, beauty, realism, dignity*), concrete nouns point to immediate, often sensory experience and to physical objects (*steeple, asphalt, lilac, stone, garlic*).

Specific, concrete nouns express meaning more vividly than general or abstract ones. Although general and abstract language is sometimes necessary to convey your meaning, ordinarily prefer specific, concrete alternatives.

▶ The senator spoke about the challenges of the future: ~~the environment and world peace.~~ *famine, pollution, dwindling resources, and terrorism.*

Nouns such as *thing, area, factor,* and *individual* are especially dull and imprecise.

▶ A career in city planning offers many ~~things.~~
    _{rewards.}

▶ Try pairing a trainee with an ~~individual with technical experience.~~
    _{experienced technician.}

W5-c Do not misuse words.

If a word is not in your active vocabulary, you may find yourself misusing it, sometimes with embarrassing consequences. When in doubt, check the dictionary.

▶ The fans were ~~migrating~~ up the bleachers in search of good seats.
    _{climbing}

▶ The Internet has so ~~diffused~~ our culture that it touches all

segments of society.
    _{permeated}

Be especially alert for misused word forms—using a noun such as *absence, significance,* or *persistence,* for example, when your meaning requires the adjective *absent, significant,* or *persistent.*

▶ Most dieters are not ~~persistence~~ enough to make a permanent

change in their eating habits.
    _{persistent}

ON THE WEB > dianahacker.com/writersref
Grammar exercises > Word choice > E-ex W5–1

W5-d Use standard idioms.

Idioms are speech forms that follow no easily specified rules. The English say "Maria went *to hospital,*" an idiom strange to American ears, which are accustomed to hearing *the* in front of *hospital.* Native speakers of a language seldom have problems with idioms, but prepositions sometimes cause trouble, especially when they follow certain verbs and adjectives. When in doubt, consult a good desk dictionary: Look up the word preceding the troublesome preposition.

UNIDIOMATIC	IDIOMATIC
abide with (a decision)	abide by (a decision)
according with	according to
agree to (an idea)	agree with (an idea)
angry at (a person)	angry with (a person)
capable to	capable of
comply to	comply with
desirous to	desirous of
different than (a person or thing)	different from (a person or thing)
intend on doing	intend to do
off of	off
plan on doing	plan to do
preferable than	preferable to
prior than	prior to
superior than	superior to
sure and	sure to
try and	try to
type of a	type of

ESL Because idioms follow no particular rules, you must learn them individually. You may find it helpful to keep a list of idioms that you frequently encounter in your reading. For idiomatic combinations of adjectives and prepositions (such as *afraid of*), see E5-c. For idiomatic combinations of verbs and prepositions (such as *search for*), see E5-d.

ON THE WEB > dianahacker.com/writersref
Grammar exercises > Word choice > E-ex W5–2

W5-e Do not rely heavily on clichés.

The pioneer who first announced that he had "slept like a log" no doubt amused his companions with a fresh and unlikely comparison. Today, however, that comparison is a cliché, a saying that has lost its dazzle from overuse. No longer can it surprise.

To see just how predictable clichés are, put your hand over the right-hand column on the next page and then finish the phrases given on the left.

cool as a	cucumber
beat around	the bush
blind as a	bat
busy as a	bee, beaver
crystal	clear
dead as a	doornail
out of the frying pan and	into the fire
light as a	feather
like a bull	in a china shop
playing with	fire
nutty as a	fruitcake
selling like	hotcakes
starting out at the bottom	of the ladder
water under the	bridge
white as a	sheet, ghost
avoid clichés like the	plague

The cure for clichés is frequently simple: Just delete them. When this won't work, try adding some element of surprise. One student, for example, who had written that she had butterflies in her stomach, revised her cliché like this:

> If all of the action in my stomach is caused by butterflies, there must be a horde of them, with horseshoes on.

The image of butterflies wearing horseshoes is fresh and unlikely, not dully predictable like the original cliché.

ON THE WEB > dianahacker.com/writersref
Language Debates > Clichés

W5-f Use figures of speech with care.

A figure of speech is an expression that uses words imaginatively (rather than literally) to make abstract ideas concrete. Most often, figures of speech compare two seemingly unlike things to reveal surprising similarities.

In a *simile,* the writer makes the comparison explicitly, usually by introducing it with *like* or *as:* "By the time cotton had to be picked, grandfather's neck was as red as the clay he plowed." In a *metaphor,* the *like* or *as* is omitted, and the comparison is implied.

For example, in the Old Testament Song of Solomon, a young woman compares the man she loves to a fruit tree: "With great delight I sat in his shadow, and his fruit was sweet to my taste."

Although figures of speech are useful devices, writers sometimes use them without thinking through the images they evoke. The result is sometimes a *mixed metaphor*, the combination of two or more images that don't make sense together.

> ▶ Crossing Utah's salt flats in his new convertible, my father flew *at jet speed.*
> ~~under a full head of steam.~~
>   ^

Flew suggests an airplane, while *under a full head of steam* suggests a steamboat or a train. To clarify the image, the writer should stick with one comparison or the other.

> ▶ Our office had decided to put all controversial issues on a back
>
> burner.~~in a holding pattern.~~
>   ^

Here the writer is mixing stoves and airplanes. Simply deleting one of the images corrects the problem.

ON THE WEB > dianahacker.com/writersref
Grammar exercises > Word choice > E-ex W5–3

W6

The dictionary and thesaurus

W6-a The dictionary

A good dictionary, whether print or online—such as *The American Heritage Dictionary of the English Language, The Random House College Dictionary, Merriam-Webster's Collegiate Dictionary,* or *Webster's New World Dictionary of the American Language*—is an indispensable writer's aid.

The entry on page 157 is taken from *The American Heritage Dictionary.* Labels show where various kinds of information about a word can be found in that dictionary. A sample entry from an online dictionary, *Merriam-Webster Online,* appears on page 158.

PRINT DICTIONARY ENTRY

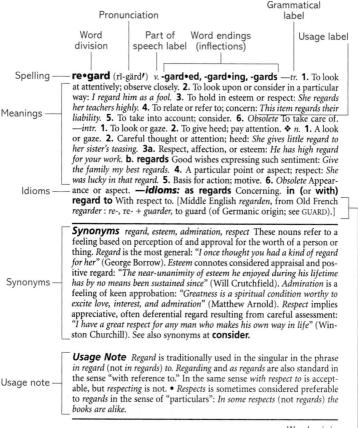

Pronunciation

Grammatical label

Word division

Part of speech label

Word endings (inflections)

Usage label

Spelling — **re•gard** (rĭ-gärd′) *v.* **-gard•ed, -gard•ing, -gards** —*tr.* **1.** To look at attentively; observe closely. **2.** To look upon or consider in a particular way: *I regard him as a fool.* **3.** To hold in esteem or respect: *She regards her teachers highly.* **4.** To relate or refer to; concern: *This item regards their liability.* **5.** To take into account; consider. **6.** *Obsolete* To take care of. —*intr.* **1.** To look or gaze. **2.** To give heed; pay attention. ❖ *n.* **1.** A look or gaze. **2.** Careful thought or attention; heed: *She gives little regard to her sister's teasing.* **3a.** Respect, affection, or esteem: *He has high regard for your work.* **b. regards** Good wishes expressing such sentiment: *Give the family my best regards.* **4.** A particular point or aspect; respect: *She was lucky in that regard.* **5.** Basis for action; motive. **6.** *Obsolete* Appearance or aspect. —***idioms:*** **as regards** Concerning. **in (or with) regard to** With respect to. [Middle English *regarden*, from Old French *regarder* : *re-*, re- + *guarder*, to guard (of Germanic origin; see GUARD).]

Meanings

Idioms

Synonyms — **Synonyms** *regard, esteem, admiration, respect* These nouns refer to a feeling based on perception of and approval for the worth of a person or thing. *Regard* is the most general: *"I once thought you had a kind of regard for her"* (George Borrow). *Esteem* connotes considered appraisal and positive regard: *"The near-unanimity of esteem he enjoyed during his lifetime has by no means been sustained since"* (Will Crutchfield). *Admiration* is a feeling of keen approbation: *"Greatness is a spiritual condition worthy to excite love, interest, and admiration"* (Matthew Arnold). *Respect* implies appreciative, often deferential regard resulting from careful assessment: *"I have a great respect for any man who makes his own way in life"* (Winston Churchill). See also synonyms at **consider.**

Usage note — **Usage Note** *Regard* is traditionally used in the singular in the phrase *in regard* (not *in regards*) *to*. *Regarding* and *as regards* are also standard in the sense "with reference to." In the same sense *with respect to* is acceptable, but *respecting* is not. • *Respects* is sometimes considered preferable to *regards* in the sense of "particulars": *In some respects* (not *regards*) *the books are alike.*

Word origin (etymology)

Spelling, word division, and pronunciation

The main entry (*re•gard* in the sample entries) shows the correct spelling of the word. When there are two correct spellings of a word (as in *collectible, collectable,* for example), both are given, with the preferred spelling usually appearing first.

The main entry also shows how the word is divided into syllables. The dot between *re* and *gard* separates the word's two syllables. When a word is compound, the main entry shows how to write it: as one word (*crossroad*), as a hyphenated word (*cross-stitch*), or as two words (*cross section*).

ONLINE DICTIONARY ENTRY

Merriam-Webster Online Dictionary

Thesaurus

3 entries found for **regard**.
To select an entry, click on it.

Alternative entries ——— regard[1.noun] Go
regard[2.verb]
self-regard

Audio pronunciation link

Spelling and word division ———

Main Entry: **¹re·gard** ◄)) Etymology
Pronunciation ——— Pronunciation: ri-ˈgärd (word origin)
Part of speech label ——— Function: *noun*
Etymology: Middle English, from Middle
Usage label ——— French, from Old French, from *regarder*
1 *archaic* : APPEARANCE
2 a : ATTENTION, CONSIDERATION <due
regard should be given to all facets of the
question> **b** : a protective interest : CARE
<ought to have more *regard* for his health>
3 : LOOK, GAZE
4 a : the worth or estimation in which
something or someone is held <a man of
Meanings (synonyms ——— small *regard*> **b** (1) : a feeling of respect and
shown as hyperlinks) affection : ESTEEM <his hard work won him
the *regard* of his colleagues> (2) *plural* :
friendly greetings implying such feeling <give
him my *regards*>
5 : a basis of action or opinion : MOTIVE
6 : an aspect to be taken into consideration :
RESPECT <is a small school, and is fortunate
in this *regard*>
7 *obsolete* : INTENTION
- **in regard to** : with respect to :
Idioms ——— CONCERNING
- **with regard to** : in regard to

The word's pronunciation is given just after the main entry. The accents indicate which syllables are stressed; the other marks are explained in the dictionary's pronunciation key. In print dictionaries this key usually appears at the bottom of every page or every other page. Many online entries include an audio link to a person's voice pronouncing the word. And most online dictionaries have an audio pronunciation guide.

Word endings and grammatical labels

When a word takes endings to indicate grammatical functions (called *inflections*), the endings are listed in boldface, as with *-garded, -garding,* and *-gards* in the sample print entry.

Labels for the parts of speech and for other grammatical terms are sometimes abbreviated, as they are in the print entry. The most commonly used abbreviations are these:

n.	noun	adj.	adjective
pl.	plural	adv.	adverb
sing.	singular	pron.	pronoun
v.	verb	prep.	preposition
tr.	transitive verb	conj.	conjunction
int.	intransitive verb	interj.	interjection

Meanings, word origin, synonyms, and antonyms

Each meaning for the word is given a number. Occasionally a word's use is illustrated in a quoted sentence.

Sometimes a word can be used as more than one part of speech (*regard,* for instance, can be used as either a verb or a noun). In such a case, all the meanings for one part of speech are given before all the meanings for another, as in the sample entries. The entries also give idiomatic uses of the word.

The origin of the word, called its *etymology,* appears in brackets after all the meanings in the print version; in the online version, it appears before the meanings.

Synonyms, words similar in meaning to the main entry, are frequently listed. In the sample print entry, the dictionary draws distinctions in meaning among the various synonyms. In the online entry, synonyms appear as hyperlinks. Antonyms, which do not appear in the sample entries, are words having a meaning opposite from that of the main entry.

Usage

Usage labels indicate when, where, or under what conditions a particular meaning for a word is appropriately used. Common labels are *informal* (or *colloquial*), *slang, nonstandard, dialect, obsolete, archaic, poetic,* and *British.* In the sample print entry, two meanings of *regard* are labeled *obsolete* because they are no longer in use. The online entry has meanings labeled both *archaic* and *obsolete.*

Dictionaries sometimes include usage notes as well. In the sample print entry, the dictionary offers advice on several uses of *regard* not specifically covered by the meanings. Such advice is based on the opinions of many experts and on actual usage in current magazines, newspapers, and books.

W6-b　The thesaurus

When you are looking for just the right word, you may want to consult a book of synonyms and antonyms such as *Roget's International Thesaurus* (or its online equivalent). Look up (or click on) the adjective *still,* for example, and you will find synonyms such as *tranquil, quiet, quiescent, reposeful, calm, pacific, halcyon, placid,* and *unruffled.* Unless your vocabulary is better than average, the list will contain words you've never heard of or with which you are only vaguely familiar. Whenever you are tempted to use one of these words, look it up in the dictionary first to avoid misusing it.

On discovering the thesaurus, many writers use it for the wrong reasons, so a word of caution is in order. Do not turn to a thesaurus in search of exotic, fancy words — such as *halcyon* — with which to embellish your essays. Look instead for words that express your meaning exactly. Most of the time these words will be familiar to both you and your readers. The first synonym on the list — *tranquil* — was probably the word you were looking for all along.